P-450 AND
CHEMICAL CARCINOGENESIS

GANN Monograph on Cancer Research

The "GANN Monograph on Cancer Research" series is promoted by the Japanese Cancer Association. This semiannual series of monographs was initiated in 1966 by the late Dr. Tomizo Yoshida (1903–1973) and is now published jointly by Japan Scientific Societies Press, Tokyo and Plenum Press, New York and London. Each volume consists of collected contributions on current topics in cancer problems and allied research fields. The publication of these monographs owes much to the financial support given by the late Professor Kazushige Higuchi, the Jikei University School of Medicine.

The planning for each volume is done by the Board of Executive Directors of the Japanese Cancer Association, with the final approval of the Board of Directors. It is hoped that the series will serve as an important source of information in the field of cancer research.

Japanese Cancer Association

JAPANESE CANCER ASSOCIATION
GANN Monograph on Cancer Research No.30

P-450 AND
CHEMICAL CARCINOGENESIS

Edited by YUSAKU TAGASHIRA
TSUNEO OMURA

JAPAN SCIENTIFIC SOCIETIES PRESS, Tokyo
PLENUM PRESS, New York and London

March 1985

Published jointly by

Japan Scientific Societies Press
2-10 Hongo, 6-chome, Bunkyo-ku, Tokyo 113, Japan
ISBN 4-7622-8433-5
          and
Plenum Press
233 Spring, Street, New York, NY 10013, USA

Distributed in all areas outside Japan and Asia between Pakistan and Korea by Plenum Press, New York and London.

Printed in Japan

PREFACE

This book is one of a GANN Monograph on Cancer Research series and is based on a Japanese Cancer Association-sponsored symposium entitled "Multiplicity of Chemical Carcinogen-Activating Enzymes with Particular Emphasis on Cytochrome P-450" which was held in Tokyo on November 21, 1983.

The principal role of microsomal cytochrome P-450 in the metabolic activation of various chemical carcinogens in animal cells has been well established. The activated chemical carcinogens induce mutations of the cells, which is an essential part of the initiation of chemical carcinogenesis. Since microsomal cytochrome P-450 in various animal tissues includes multiple molecular species with different substrate specificities and different responses to chemical inducers, knowledge of the molecular and catalytic properties and the inducibilities of those cytochrome P-450 forms is surely a most important base from which to elucidate the mechanism of chemical carcinogenesis.

The focus of the symposium was this area of molecular diversity and inducibility of microsomal cytochrome P-450 in animal tissues. The mechanism of activation of various types of chemical carcinogens by cytochrome P-450 and related enzymes was another main topic. The editors, who were also the symposium organizers, hope these summaries of current research in this field in Japan will stimulate future development of studies on the mechanism of chemical carcinogenesis.

February 1985

Yusaku TAGASHIRA
Tsuneo OMURA

INTRODUCTION

Yusaku Tagashira[*1] and Tsuneo Omura[*2]

*[*1]Department of Biochemistry, Saitama Cancer Center Research Institute,
and *[*2]Department of Biology, Faculty of Science, Kyushu University*

Since the first memorable success of Yamagiwa and Ichikawa in the mid-1910's in producing experimental carcinomas in rabbits by applying coal tar to the ears of the animals (*21, 22*), numerous chemical compounds have been shown to induce tumors in experimental animals. However, many of those carcinogenic chemical compounds including polycyclic aromatic hydrocarbons were rather chemically inert, and the mechanism of their action on animal tissue cells remained unknown until recently. The metabolism of these compounds in animals was studied and many of them were found to be oxidatively metabolized in the liver. However, the oxidative enzyme system in the liver, which was supposed to be involved in such metabolism, was quite unstable. Its nature also remained unclear until the beginning of the 1960's, when the discovery and characterization of cytochrome P-450 in liver microsomes (*16, 17*) and the finding of its participation in the oxidative metabolism of steroids and various xenobiotic compounds (*2, 4*) opened a way to solve the question of how the carcinogenic chemical compounds affect animal cells to induce their malignant transformations.

In early studies on the physiological functions of cytochrome P-450, attention was focused on its role in the "detoxication" of various synthetic drugs in animals, since the oxidative metabolism it catalyzed in microsomes was found to be an essential initial step for the excretion of many lipophilic drugs from animals as water-soluble conjugates. However, it was also found that the toxicity of some chemical compounds was apparently potentiated by the oxidative metabolisms in animal bodies. The contribution of cytochrome P-450 to the manifestation of the cytotoxic effects of some chemical carcinogens was suspected, and by the end of the 1960's was confirmed. Polycyclic aromatic hydrocarbons including benzo(a)pyrene are not cytotoxic in themselves but become highly cytotoxic when metabolized by the cytochrome P-450 enzyme system (*6*).

Studies on the oxidative metabolism of aromatic hydrocarbons by microsomal cytochrome P-450 led to the conclusion that the primary products of the oxidation reaction were arene oxides (*14*), which were then transformed to phenols, dihydrodiols, or various conjugates by non-enzymatic or enzymatic reactions. The primary microsomal oxidation products of carcinogenic aromatic hydrocarbons were also their arene oxides (*8, 19*), which were reactive enough to combine with proteins and nucleic acids (*5, 7*). In addition to the aromatic hydrocarbons, many other carcinogenic xenobiotic compounds were also oxidatively metabolized by microsomal cytochrome P-450 to react with nuclear deoxyribonucleic acid to disturb the genetic information of the cells

[*1] Komuro 818, Ina-machi, Kitaadachi-gun, Saitama 362, Japan (田頭勇作).

[*2] Hakozaki 6-10-1, Higashi-ku, Fukuoka 812, Japan (大村恒雄).

(*12*). This important understanding of the mechanism of action of various chemical carcinogens on animal cells led Ames *et al.* (*1*) to establish a new simple test system for the detection of potential mutagens to animals.

A wide variety of synthetic chemical compounds are oxidized by the cytochrome P-450 enzyme system of liver microsomes. Initial attempts by biochemists to purify this substance from liver microsomes to solve the problem of this unusually broad substrate specificity of the enzyme system were hampered by the instability of microsomal cytochrome P-450 to solubilization treatments. However, an important discovery by Ichikawa and Yamano (*13*) concerning the stabilization of solubilized cytochrome P-450 by polyols and thiol compounds was a break-through in the purification of microsomal cytochrome P-450. By the middle of the 1970's, several different forms of cytochrome P-450 had been purified from liver microsomes (*10, 11, 18*), and the multiple molecular nature of microsomal cytochrome P-450 in various types of animal cells was firmly established.

It was also found that the relative amounts of those multiple forms of the substance in liver microsomes changed greatly when the animals were treated with certain types of chemical compounds (*9, 20*). Since different forms of cytochrome P-450 showed different substrate specificities, its isozyme composition in the microsomes and their alteration by the administration of xenobiotic compounds to animals determine the metabolism of these latter compounds in the cells of animal tissues. Various forms of cytochrome P-450 produce different metabolites from benzo(a)pyrene, resulting in significant difference in the binding of the metabolites to DNA (*3*). Different forms of cytochrome P-450 contribute differently to the activation of chemical carcinogens, as judged from their mutagenic activities in the Ames' test (*15*). Analysis of the isozyme composition of cytochrome P-450 in microsomes is essential when the activation of chemical carcinogens in an animal tissue is to be examined.

Studies on the purification and characterization of the multiple forms of cytochrome P-450 in microsomes from various animal tissues have made significant progress in the past several years. The cloning and analysis of cytochrome P-450 genes are also being intensively studied. Since the essential role of cytochrome P-450 in the initiation of chemical carcinogenesis in animals is now clearly established, further studies on the substance and its participation in the metabolism and activation of carcinogenic xenobiotic compounds will undoubtedly make a great contribution to the elucidation of the mechanism of chemical carcinogenesis in human tissues as well as in experimental animals.

REFERENCES

1. Ames, B. N., Durston, W. E., Yamasaki, E., and Lee, F. D. Carcinogens are mutagens: A simple system combining liver homogenate for activation and bacteria for detection. *Proc. Natl. Acad. Sci. U.S.A.*, **70**, 2281–2285 (1973).
2. Cooper, D. Y., Levin, S., Narasimhulu, S., Rosenthal, O., and Estabrook, R. W. Photochemical action spectrum of the terminal oxidase of mixed function oxidase system. *Science*, **147**, 400–402 (1965).
3. Deutsch, J., Leutz, J. C., Yang, S. K., Gelboin, H. V., Chiang, Y. L., Vatsis, K. P., and Coon, M. J. Regio- and stereoselectivity of various forms of purified cytochrome P-450 in the metabolism of benzo(a)pyrene and (−)trans-7,8-dihydroxy-7,8-dihydrobenzo(a)-

pyrene as shown by product formation and binding to DNA. *Proc. Natl. Acad. Sci. U.S.A.*, **75**, 3123–3127 (1978).

4. Estabrook, R. W., Cooper, D. Y., and Rosenthal, O. The light reversible carbon monoxide inhibition of the steroid C21-hydroxylase system of the adrenal cortex. *Biochem. Z.*, **338**, 741–755 (1963).

5. Gelboin, H. V. A microsome-dependent binding of benzo(a)pyrene to DNA. *Cancer Res.*, **29**, 1272–1276 (1969).

6. Gelboin, H. V., Huberman, E., and Sachs, L. Enzymatic hydroxylation of benzopyrene and its relationship to cytotoxicity. *Proc. Natl. Acad. Sci. U.S.A.*, **64**, 1188–1194 (1969).

7. Grover, P. L. and Sims, P. Enzyme-catalyzed reactions of polycyclic hydrocarbons with deoxyribonucleic acid and protein *in vitro*. *Biochem. J.*, **110**, 159–160 (1969).

8. Grover, P. L., Hewer, A., and Sims, P. Epoxides as microsomal metabolities of polycyclic hydrocarbons. *FEBS Lett.*, **18**, 76–80 (1971).

9. Harada, N. and Omura, T. Selective induction of two different molecular species of cytochrome P-450 by phenobarbital and 3-methylcholanthrene. *J. Biochem.*, **89**, 237–248 (1981).

10. Hashimoto, C. and Imai, Y. Purification of a substrate complex of cytochrome P-450 from liver microsomes of 3-methylcholanthrene-treated rabbits. *Biochem. Biophys. Res. Commun.*, **68**, 821–827 (1976).

11. Haugen, D. A., Hoeven, T. A., and Coon, M. J. Purified liver microsomal cytochrome P-450. Separation and characterization of multiple forms. *J. Biol. Chem.*, **250**, 3567–3570 (1975).

12. Heidelberger, C. Chemical carcinogenesis. *Annu. Rev. Biochem.*, **44**, 79–119 (1975).

13. Ichikawa, Y. and Yamano, T. Reconversion of detergent- and sulfhydryl reagent-produced P-420 to P-450 by polyols and glutathione. *Biochim. Biophys. Acta*, **131**, 490–497 (1967).

14. Jerina, D. M., Daly, J. W., Witkop, B., Zaltman-Nirenberg, P., and Udenfriend, S. 1,2-Naphthalene oxide as an intermediate in the microsomal hydroxylation of naphthalene. *Biochemistry*, **9**, 147–155 (1970).

15. Kawajiri, K., Yonekawa, H., Harada, N., Noshiro, M., Omura, T., and Tagashira, Y. Immunochemical study on the role of different types of microsomal cytochrome P-450 in mutagenesis by chemical carcinogens. *Cancer Res.*, **40**, 1652–1657 (1980).

16. Omura, T. and Sato, R. A new cytochrome in liver microsomes. *J. Biol. Chem.*, **237**, 1375–1376 (1962).

17. Omura, T. and Sato, R. The carbon monoxide-binding Pigment of liver microsomes. I. Evidence for its hemoprotein nature. *J. Biol. Chem.*, **239**, 2370–2378 (1964).

18. Ryan, D., Lu, A.Y.H., Kawalek J., West, S. B., and Levin, W. Highly purified cytochrome P-448 and P-450 from rat liver microsomes. *Biochem. Biophys. Res. Commun.*, **64**, 1134–1141 (1975).

19. Silkirk, J. K., Huberman, E., and Heidelberger, C. An epoxide is an intermediate in the microsomal metabolism of the chemical carcinogens, dibenz(a, h)anthracene. *Biochem. Biophys. Res. Commun.*, **43**, 1010–1016 (1971).

20. Thomas, P. E., Korzeniowsky, K., Ryan, D., and Levin, W. Preparation of monospecific antibodies against two forms of rat liver cytochrome P-450 and quantitation of these antigens in microsomes. *Arch. Biochem. Biophys.*, **192**, 524–532 (1979).

21. Yamagiwa, K. and Ichikawa, K. Pathogenesis of carcinoma. *Gann*, **12**, 1–29 (1918).

22. Yamagiwa, K. and Ichikawa, K. Experimental study of the pathogenesis of carcinoma. *J. Cancer Res.*, **3**, 1–29 (1918).

CONTENTS

MOLECULAR MULTIPLICITY
OF CYTOCHROME P-450

GANN Monograph on Cancer Research 30, 1985

PHYSICOCHEMICAL PROPERTIES OF MULTIPLE FORMS OF CYTOCHROME P-450: A PROPOSAL FOR THE LIGAND STRUCTURE

Yuzo Yoshida

*Faculty of Pharmaceutical Sciences, Mukogawa University**

Cytochrome P-450 is characterized by unique molecular spectroscopic properties such as the unusually red-shifted Soret band of its reduced CO complex. These spectral properties are due to the ligation of thiolate (S^-) of cysteine at the fifth coordination position of the heme iron. The sixth ligand *trans* to thiolate of this cytochrome is exchangeable as suggested by the occurrence of substrate-induced spectral change. Its most likely candidate is a water molecule and the water-ligated form may be a low-spin complex. Hydrophobicity of the heme crevice probably acts as a barrier keeping the water molecule from access to the heme iron, and the cytochrome seems to be in an equilibrium between the water-ligated (low-spin) and water-dissociated (high-spin) forms. The equilibrium is thought to be affected by the hydrophobicity of the heme crevice. This hydrophobicity may differ in molecular species and be altered by substrate binding. The occurrence of molecular species with different spin states and different substrate- or temperature-dependent spin state changes, particular peculiarities of cytochrome P-450, can both be explained by the ligand structure described above.

Since the rediscovery of cytochrome P-450 as a protoheme protein by Omura and Sato (*24, 25*), this material has attracted the attention of many biophysicists because of its unique spectral characteristics. The most outstanding and best-known feature is the unusually red-shifted Soret band of the reduced CO complex occurring in the 450-nm region. Upon denaturation by various treatments, the cytochrome loses this unique spectral property as well as its catalytic activity (*14, 18, 24, 25*). Spectral properties of the reduced CO complex of the denatured form called "P-420" (*24, 25*) are identical to those of ordinary protoheme proteins such as myoglobin and hemoglobin. These facts indicate that the unusual spectral properties of cytochrome P-450 closely relate to its function. The many efforts made to elucidate the structural bases of these unique spectral characteristics have revealed that they are predominantly due to thiolate (S^-) ligation at the fifth coordination position (*3, 6, 8, 20, 21, 26, 30, 31*).

While, it is well-known that there are many molecular species of cytochrome P-450 which show a wide variety of catalytic properties (*9*). Although a few differences are observed in their physicochemical properties, no satisfying physicochemical explanation is available for this multiplicity. This paper focuses on a brief description of the spectral characteristics of cytochrome P-450 in relation to the ligand structure.

---

* Edagawacho 4-16, Nishinomiya, Hyogo 663, Japan (吉田雄三).

Spectral and Magnetic Characteristics of Cytochrome P-450

Figure 1 shows the absorption spectra of two typical species of cytochrome P-450, called P-450 LM$_2$ *(13)* or P-450$_1$ *(17)* (A) and P-450 LM$_4$ *(13)* or P-448$_1$ *(17)* (B), occurring in rabbit liver microsomes. The most striking and best-known spectral feature of the cytochrome is the red-shifted Soret band of the reduced CO complex. Other characteristics are: 1) In the oxidized state, the cytochrome can occur in either high- or low-spin forms; LM$_2$ (Fig. 1A) and LM$_4$ (Fig. 1B) represent the low-spin and the high-spin forms, respectively; 2) the α band of the ferric low-spin form is observed as a distinct peak at 570 nm (Fig. 1A), whereas those of many other ordinary ferric low-spin protoheme proteins are observed as shoulders on their β bands; 3) the Soret band of the reduced form is unusual with respect to its position and intensity.

The electron paramagnetic resonance (EPR) spectrum of the ferric low-spin cytochrome P-450 shows the characteristic triplet signals at $g=1.91$, 2.25, and 2.41, termed g_x, g_y, and g_z, respectively *(15)*. This characteristic set corresponds to those of "microsomal Fe$_x$" *(11)* found in rabbit liver microsomes early in the investigation on microsomal redox systems. Although triplet signals are a common feature of EPR spectra of many low-spin heme proteins, the narrow separation between g_x and g_z is

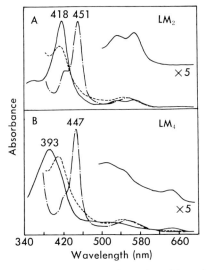

FIG. 1.   Absorption spectra of two typical species of hepatic microsomal cytochrome P-450. A: cytochrome P-450 LM$_2$ *(13)*. B: cytochrome P-450 LM$_4$ *(13)*.
——— oxidized form; - - - - reduced form; —·— reduced CO complex.

TABLE I.   EPR Parameters of Cytochromes P-450 and b_5 and Metmyoglobin Derivatives *(20)*

Hemoproteins	g_z	g_y	g_x
Cytochrome P-450	2.42	2.25	1.92
Metmyoglobin-thiol	2.39	2.24	1.94
Cytochrome b_5	3.03	2.23	1.43
Metmyoglobin-imidazole	2.86	2.27	1.53

characteristic of cytochrome P-450 (Table I). So, the EPR spectrum is a convenient index of this cytochrome together with the reduced CO difference spectrum (15).

Identification of Thiolate as the Fifth Ligand

In 1978, Chang and Dolphin (3) synthesized ferrous protoporphyrin IX dimethyl ester coordinated with some alkylthiolate-crown ether complexes. Soret bands of these complexes appeared at 408 nm and were shifted to 451 nm upon addition of CO, suggesting that their ligand structure was close to that of cytochrome P-450. A few model complexes (8, 21, 31) that could mimic the spectral properties of cytochrome P-450 were also developed. The most important structural feature commonly observed in these complexes was the presence of thiolate at the fifth coordination position of the heme iron. Absorption spectra of other complexes without thiolate were reported to be different from that of cytochrome P-450 (3, 8, 21, 31). These facts suggested that the unique spectral characteristics of cytochrome P-450 were due to the thiolate ligation.

The similarity of thiolate ligated protoheme derivatives to cytochrome P-450 was also supported by their EPR spectra (4, 20). For example, g values of metmyoglobin coordinated by propanethiol ($g_x=1.94$, $g_y=2.24$, $g_z=2.39$) were close to those of ferric low-spin cytochrome P-450, whereas the imidazole complex of metmyoglobin showed g_x, g_y, and g_z at 1.53, 2.27, and 2.86, respectively, values comparable to those of cytochrome b_5 (Table I) (20).

In addition to these spectral and EPR studies, recent resonance Raman (26) and magnetic circular dichroism (CD) (30) analysis of cytochromes P-450 suggested the high basicity or strong electron-donating character of the axial ligand. Proton nuclear magnetic resonance (NMR) of ferric cytochrome P-450 suggested the presence of a ligand with strong field at the fifth coordination position of the heme iron (15). These observations coincide with the concept that one of the axial ligands is thiolate. The confirming evidence for the thiolate ligation at the fifth coordination position was obtained from an analysis with extended X-ray absorption fine structure (EXAFS) spectroscopy of P-450 LM$_2$ (Fig. 2) (6).

Based on these lines of evidence, it is now established that the fifth ligand of cytochrome P-450 is thiolate of a cysteinyl residue of the apoprotein, and this is considered to be the most important structural feature of the cytochrome.

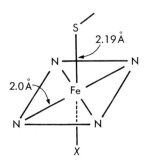

Fig. 2. Ligand structure of P-450 LM$_2$ deduced from the data of EXAFS spectroscopy (6).

Substrate-induced Spectral Change: Properties Related to Sixth Ligand

Ferric cytochrome P-450 is known to change its absorption spectrum upon binding with substrates and related organic compounds (*19, 28*). Such spectral change is usually classified into three categories, type I, type II, and modified type II (or reverse type I) (Fig. 3) (*28*). The mechanisms of each type were extensively studied by Yoshida and Kumaoka (*34*) and the following conclusions were drawn. 1) Type I spectral change represents the low to high spin state change of the cytochrome due to removal or exchange of the endogenous sixth ligand caused by the binding with a hydrophobic molecule. 2) Type II spectral change is due to replacement of an internal sixth ligand with an amino group in an added compound. 3) Modified type II (or reverse type I) spectral change is due to binding of a hydroxyl group in an added compound to the sixth coordination position of the high-spin form. Although the mechanisms inducing these spectral changes differ, they are uniformly dependent on the high movability of the endogenous sixth ligand. In general, the sixth coordination position of a low-spin protoheme protein is usually occupied by a relatively strong internal ligand which cannot be easily removed or replaced by an exogenously added compound, though that of a high-spin one can readily be replaced by some external compounds. The high movability of the sixth ligand of ferric low-spin form is therefore probably a characteristic of cytochrome P-450.

Evidence for Oxygen Ligation at the Sixth Coordination Position of Ferric Low-spin Cytochrome P-450

On the sixth ligand *trans* to thiolate of ferric low-spin cytochrome P-450, two contrary concepts have been proposed. Chevion *et al.* (*4*) deduced that the sixth ligand was imidazole of a histidine moiety in the apoprotein by examining the EPR data of various cytochromes P-450 and their model complexes using the crystal field theory.

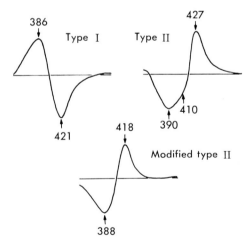

Fɪɢ. 3.   Schematic representation of three distinctive types of substrate-induced difference spectrum of hepatic microsomal cytochrome P-450.

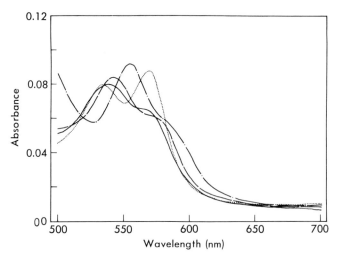

Fig. 4.   Absorption spectra of ferric P-450$_1$ and its derivatives (33). - - - - native form; —— 1-methylimidazole complex; —— pyridine complex; —·— KCN complex.

In contrast, Griffin and Peterson (10) suggested the presence of a water molecule at the sixth coordination position of the ferric low-spin form based on the measurement of spin relaxation rate of water protons by means of pulse NMR technique.

Recently, another spectrophotometric approach to identifying the native sixth ligand of the ferric low-spin form has been made independently by us (33) and two other groups (7, 32). We (33) used two species of cytochrome P-450 purified from rabbit liver microsomes; one was a low-spin form called P-450$_1$ (17) which is the same as P-450 LM$_2$ (13) (Fig. 1A), and the other was a high-spin one called P-448$_1$ (17) corresponding to P-450 LM$_4$ (13) (Fig. 1B). As shown in Fig. 1A, the conspicuous α band is characteristic of ferric low-spin cytochrome P-450. This characteristic was, however, lost upon binding with an exogenous ligand such as 1-methylimidazole, pyridine or cyanide (Fig. 4) (33). Since binding of these ligands did not denature P-450$_1$ to P-420 under the experimental conditions, they did not replace the fifth ligand, thiolate, but did the sixth one, *trans* to thiolate (33). So, the conspicuous α band of the native low-spin form of the cytochrome must reflect the nature of the endogenous sixth ligand. Thus, the native sixth ligand of the ferric low-spin cytochrome P-450 can be assumed if the characteristic shape of its absorption spectrum is mimicked by a certain cytochrome P-450 derivative bound with a known compound as the sixth ligand.

As shown in Fig. 4, the conspicuous α band was not observed in the absorption spectra of P-450$_1$ derivatives bound with imidazole and pyridine. This suggests that the native sixth ligand of the ferric low-spin cytochrome P-450 is different from these nitrogenous ones (33). We next made comparable experiments with P-448$_1$ (33). This species is usually in a high-spin state without substrate (12) and is considered to have a very weak ligand or none at all at the sixth coordination position. As shown in Fig. 5, P-448$_1$ shows an absorption spectrum characteristic for high-spin ferric form showing two charge transfer bands at about 500 and 650 nm. Upon binding with some nitrogenous bases such as pyridine and 1-methylimidazole, P-448$_1$ converted to a low-spin

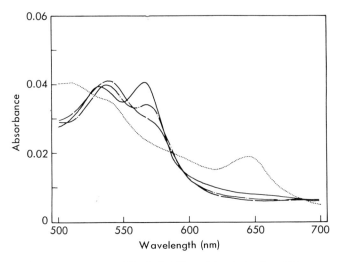

FIG. 5. Absorption spectra of ferric P-448₁ and its derivatives (*33*). - - - - native form; —— pyridine complex; —·— 2-methylpyridine complex; —— 1-propanol complex.

complex having α and β bands (Fig. 5, spectrum of 1-methylimidazole complex is not shown). Absorption spectra of these complexes were practically superimposable on the corresponding ones derived from P-450₁ (Fig. 4), indicating that P-448₁ shows essentially the same spectrum as P-450₁ when their sixth coordination position are occupied by the same ligand. In this context, the absorption spectrum of the 2-methyl-pyridine complex of P-448₁ is noteworthy. As can be seen in Fig. 5, α band of this complex is more conspicuous than that of the pyridine complex. Essentially the same relationship was observed also between the absorption spectra of 1-methylimidazole and 2-methylimidazole complexes of P-448₁ (data not shown). The ligand fields of 2-methylpyridine and 2-methylimidazole are respectively weaker than those of pyridine and 1-methylimidazole, because of the steric hinderance by the methyl groups adjacent to their coordinating nitrogen atoms. It can thus be deduced that the relative intensity of α bands of ferric low-spin derivatives of cytochrome P-450 are inversely proportional to the field strength of their sixth ligands. Consequently, the sixth ligand of the native low-spin cytochrome P-450 must have fairly weak field strength. As shown in Fig. 5, an alkanol such as *n*-propanol could coordinate to the heme iron of P-448₁ and formed

TABLE II. Spectral Parameters of the Soret Region of P-450₁ and P-448₁ and Their Derivatives

Ligands	P-450₁		P-448₁	
	λ_{max} (nm)	ε (mM^{-1} cm^{-1})	λ_{max} (nm)	ε (mM^{-1} cm^{-1})
Native	418	107	393	96
Pyridine	422	103	421	103
1-Methylimidazole	425	100	424	97
KCN	440	93	—	—
2-Methylpyridine	421	105	421	103
1-Propanol	—	—	417	110

a low-spin complex, though alcohols are fairly weak ligands. The intensity of α band of this complex was higher than that of the 2-methylpyridine complex and the absorption spectrum was practically superimposable on that of P-450$_1$ (Fig. 4). These observations strongly suggest that the sixth ligand of the native low-spin cytochrome P-450 is not a nitrogenous but an oxygenous one. Ligation of an oxygenous ligand was further supported by the spectral data of the Soret region. As shown in Table II, spectral parameters of Soret bands of P-450$_1$ derivatives bound with pyridine and 1-methylimidazole were practically the same as those of the corresponding P-448$_1$ derivatives. These peaks were located at wavelengths longer than 420 nm and showed hypochromicity compared with the Soret band of the native low-spin form of P-450$_1$. On the other hand, n-alkanols bound only to P-448$_1$ and the spectral data of the Soret band of the n-propanol complex of P-448$_1$ (Table II) were practically identical with those of the native P-450$_1$.

According to traditional concepts, oxygenous compounds such as water and alcohols are weak ligands and ferric protoheme proteins ligated by them are usually in a high-spin state. Actually, many ferric protoheme proteins such as hemoglobin, myoglobin, and peroxidases whose relationship between their ligand structure and spectral properties has been extensively studied are in high-spin state when they bind with an oxygenous ligand. Occurrence of an oxygenous ligand at the sixth coordination position of native low-spin form of cytochrome P-450 seems curious. Thus, there are other proposals that the sixth ligand may be nitrogenous, such as the histidine residue of apoprotein though the field strength of the ligand may be weakened by steric factors (29). However, absorption spectra of the nitrogen-ligated forms of P-450$_1$ and P-448$_1$ were clearly distinguished from that of the native low-spin form even if the field strength of an added ligand was weakened by steric hinderance as in the case of 2-methylpyridine (33) (see Figs. 4 and 5). Furthermore, the absorption spectrum of the P-448$_1$ derivative bound with 2-ethylpyridine whose ligand field was weaker than that of 2-methylpyridine was practically identical with that of the 2-methylpyridine P-448$_1$ (33). These observations seem to rule out the ligation of a sterically hindered nitrogenous ligand to the sixth coordination position of the native ferric low-spin cytochrome P-450. It can thus, be concluded that the most probable sixth ligand of the native ferric low-spin cytochrome P-450 is an oxygenous one.

Proposal of the Entity of the Oxygenous Ligand

The sixth ligand of the native low-spin ferric cytochrome P-450 has been established as oxygenous (7, 10, 32, 33), and there arises next the problem of identifying its entity. A water molecule or an oxyamino acid side chain of the apoprotein are possible candidates for the naturally occurring oxygenous ligand.

Recently, the author performed experiments to determine this entity (35). Lower alkanols such as methanol, ethanol, propanol, and butanol bound to high-spin cytochrome P-450 and converted it to a low-spin form (32–34) (see Fig. 5 and Table II). Standard free energy change ($\Delta G°$), standard entropy change ($\Delta S°$), and standard enthalpy change ($\Delta H°$) of the alkanol binding to the cytochrome in microsomes were calculated from the temperature dependency of the values of spectral K_d of alkanols (35). As shown in Figs. 6 and 7, thermodynamic parameters of the alkanol binding were

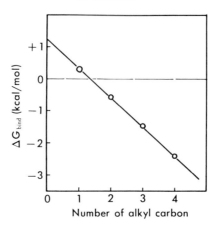

FIG. 6.   Relationship between $\Delta G°$ of alkanol binding and alkyl chain length of alkanol. Microsomes from 3-methylcholanthrene-treated rats were suspended in 0.1 M potassium phosphate buffer, pH 7.5, and titrated at 22.5° with methanol, ethanol, n-propanol, and n-butanol. Binding of an alkanol to cytochrome P-450 was determined spectrophotometrically and K_d was assumed by the usual double reciprocal plot method. $\Delta G°$ of alkanol binding was then calculated from the equation: $\Delta G° = -RT \ln (1/K_d)$.

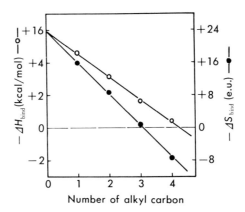

FIG. 7.   Relationship of $\Delta H°$ and $\Delta S°$ of alkanol binding to alkyl chain length of alkanol. Essentially the same experiments as Fig. 6 were performed at various temperatures and $\Delta H°$ and $\Delta S°$ were calculated from the resulting van't Hoff plots.

changed depending on the alkyl-chain length. The $\Delta G°$ was increased by -0.8 kcal/mol when one methylene unit was added to the alkyl chain (Fig. 6). This indicated that the affinity of these alkanols to the high-spin cytochrome was not limited by steric factors, because negative value of $\Delta G°$ was increased, i.e., affinity was increased, by extension of the alkyl chain. The increment of negative value of $\Delta G°$ per methylene unit was comparable to that observed in the transfer of alkyl chains from water to a hydrophobic phase (23). As shown in Fig. 7, $\Delta S°$ and $\Delta H°$ of the alkanol binding were also dependent linearly on the alkyl chain length; they were negative for methanol and were changed toward positive by the increasing alkyl chain length, indicating that the increasing affinity of alkanols to the cytochrome was dependent on the entropy change. The values of $\Delta S°$ were negative for methanol, ethanol, and propanol (nearly zero) but positive for butanol. This seems interesting because methanol, ethanol, and propanol are miscible with water but butanol is not. Based on these lines of evidence, it can be concluded that the accessibility of an alkanol to the heme site of the high-spin cytochrome is predominantly dependent on its hydrophobicity. This, in turn, suggests the presence of some hydrophobic barrier to the access of an alkanol to the sixth coordination position of the high-spin form. Recently, Backes *et al.* (*1, 2*) reported similar observations on the binding of aromatic hydrocarbons to hepatic microsomal low-spin cytochromes P-450 with a type I spectral change. Their results seem to suggest the presence of a hydrophobic barrier also to the access hydrocarbon to the substrate binding site of the low-spin form, and such a barrier is not likely to be microsomal membrane (*2*); it may be some hydrophobicity of the heme crevice including the substrate binding site. Since the substrate site of cytochrome P-450 is thought to be close to the sixth coordination position of the heme, the oxygen activation site, the hydrophobic barrier mentioned above is likely to be the same as that postulated for the alkanol binding to the high-spin form. In other words, the heme crevice of cytochrome P-450 must be hydrophobic and hydrophobicity of a compound must be an important factor in determining its accessibility to the heme site.

Upon binding with various hydrocarbons, rat liver low-spin cytochrome P-450 referred to as P-448$_2$ (P-450$_c$) is known to convert to high-spin form with type I spectral change (*16*). In this case, the extent of spin-state conversion or magnitude of the spectral change observed in the presence of a saturating concentration of an added substrate varied in substrates (*16*). This phenomenon was observed not only on purified P-448$_2$

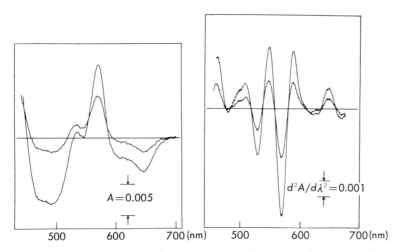

FIG. 8. Methanol-induced differences spectra of β-naphthoflavone-treated rat liver microsomes (left) and their second-derivative spectra (right). Liver microsomes from β-naphthoflavone-treated rats were suspended in 0.1 M potassium phosphate buffer, pH 7.0, containing 20% glycerol and the methanol-induced difference spectra were recorded (left). These spectra were differentiated with a Shimadzu SAPCOM-1 spectral data processor at a sampling interval of 2 nm (right).

but also on the microsomes from β-naphthoflavone-treated rats. These facts suggested that P-448$_2$ in rat liver microsomes is in the spin state equilibrium and the equilibrium is shifted to the high-spin side by binding with a substrate, the extent of the shift being dependent on the nature of the bound substrate. Then, the effects of various compounds on the binding of methanol to cytochrome P-450 in the microsomes from β-naphthoflavone-treated rats were studied (*35*). Binding of methanol to high-spin cytochrome P-450 has usually been detected by the reverse type I difference spectrum of the Soret region. However, the aromatic hydrocarbons used in these experiments as the compounds bound to P-448$_2$ showed some sharp and strong absorption peaks in this region and interfered with the detection of methanol binding by the usual method. Methanol binding was therefore detected by the spectral change in the visible region using second-drivative spectrophotometry (*35*) (Fig. 8). In the second-derivative difference spectrum, signal intensity difference ($\Delta[d^2A/d\lambda^2]$) between 570 and 548 nm (Fig. 8) was used as an index of methanol binding to the high-spin form. An apparent K_d of methanol and the maximum intensity of the difference spectrum could be calculated from the double-reciprocal plot of the signal intensity against methanol concentration. Since lower alkanols can bind to any high-spin cytochromes P-450 and convert them to low-spin complexes (*34*), the maximum intensity of the difference spectrum could be taken as an index for the content of the high-spin form

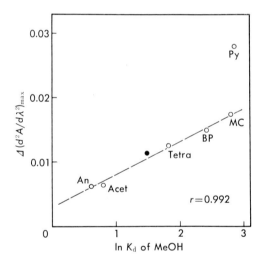

FIG. 9. Correlation between values of ln K_d of methanol and maximum intensities of the methanol-induced difference spectra of β-naphthoflavone-treated rat liver microsomes bound with various substrates. Liver microsomes from β-naphthoflavone-treated rats were suspended in 0.1 M potassium phosphate buffer, pH 7.0, containing 20% glycerol and were saturated with indicated compounds. These microsomes were titrated with methanol and binding of methanol to cytochrome P-450 was detected by second derivative spectrometry as shown in Fig. 8. K_d and maximum intensity were assumed from the usual double reciprocal plot. The compounds added were: anthrathene (An), benz[a]pyrene (BP), 3-methylcholanthrene (MC), pyrene (Py), and tetraphene (Terta). These compounds were added to the microsomal suspension as acetone solution; "Acet" indicates the samples receiving only the solvent. ● the control experiment using microsomes with no additions.

in the microsomes. Figure 9 represents the relationship between $\ln K_d$ and the maximum intensity of the methanol-induced difference spectrum ($\Delta[d^2A/d\lambda^2]$) observed in the presence of saturating amounts of indicated hydrocarbons on the β-naphthoflavone-induced microsomes. There is good correlation between these parameters. As shown in Fig. 10, a similar relationship was also observed on the microsomes from phenobarbital-treated rats. Furthermore, when the values of maximum intensity of the difference spectra were normalized with respect to cytochrome P-450 content, linear correlation between the maximum intensity and $\ln K_d$ could be observed among various microsome preparations (Fig. 11). Since the maximum intensity and $\ln K_d$ can be taken as indices for the high-spin content in the cytochrome and the free energy change of the methanol binding, respectively, these observations indicated that the accessibility of methanol to the coordination sphere of the cytochrome is inversely proportional to the high-spin content. As discussed above, the heme environment of the cytochrome is fairly hydrophobic and the accessibility of an alkanol to the heme iron is determined by their hydrophobicity rather than their bulkiness. Now, methanol is the smallest alkanol and prefers a hydrophilic environment to a hydrophobic one as indicated by the positive ΔG° of its binding to the microsomal cytochrome P-450 (Fig. 6). So, the results shown in Figs. 9–11 seem to suggest that the shift of spin state equilibrium towards high-spin is related to the increment of hydrophobicity of the heme environment.

The low to high spin state transition of cytochrome P-450 is considered to be caused by the removal of the endogenous sixth ligand of the low-spin form and this process can be expressed schematically as in Fig. 12. If the sixth ligand is a hydroxyl

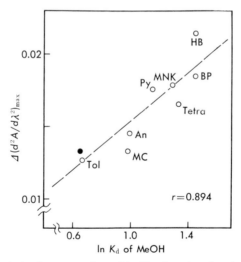

FIG. 10. Correlation between values of $\ln K_d$ of methanol and maximum intensities of the methanol-induced difference spectra of phenobarbital-treated rat liver microsomes bound with various substrates. Experiments were performed as in Fig. 9 using the microsomes from phenobarbital-treated rats. Compounds added were anthracene (An), benzo[a]pyrene (BP), hexobarbital (HB), 3-methylcholanthrene (MC), methyl n-nonyl ketone (MNK), pyrene (Py), tetraphene (Tetra), and tolene (Tol). ● the control experiment using microsomes with no additions.

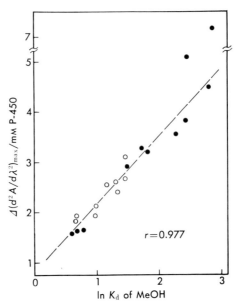

FIG. 11.   Correlation between values of $\ln K_d$ of methanol and maximum intensities of the methanol-induced difference spectra normalized with cytochrome
P-450 content. The data of Figs. 9 and 10 and of the same-type of experiments
were plotted on the same plane after normalization of the maximum intensities
with cytochrome P-450 content of each microsome preparation. $\bigcirc$, $\bullet$ the data of
phenobarbital- and β-naphthoflavone-treated microsomes, respectively.

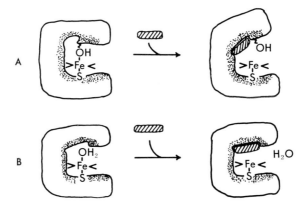

FIG. 12.   Two possible candidates for the sixth ligand of low-spin cytochrome
P-450 and their relationship to the spin state change.

group in the apoprotein, the spin state transition may require some conformation change
of the protein. In this context, the low to high spin state transition caused by the substrate binding may be due to the substrate-induced conformation change and resulting
removal of the sixth ligand (Fig. 12A). In contrast, if the endogenous sixth ligand is
a water molecule, the spin state equilibrium may reflect the binding equilibrium of
solvent water to the heme iron (Fig. 12B) and hydrophobicity of the heme environment
must affect this equilibrium. So, the substrate-induced spin state change can be ex-

plained by the change in hydrophobicity of the heme environment caused by the substrate-binding.

As described above, the heme environment of the cytochrome must be hydrophobic and the accessibility of an alkanol to the coordination sphere seems dependent on the lipophilicity of the alkanol (Figs. 6 and 7). In addition, thermodynamic analysis of methanol binding to substrate-bound cytochrome P-450 in rat liver microsomes (Figs. 9–11) indicated that the extent of low to high spin state change caused by substrate binding was related to the increment of hydrophobicity of the heme environment. These observations seem to support the presumption that the native sixth ligand of the low-spin form is a water molecule.

It is now known that some cytochrome P-450 species are in spin state equilibrium even in the presence of saturating concentrations of substrates (5, 16, 22, 27). It is hard to explain such equilibrium by the mechanism shown in Fig. 12A, because the spin state transition is coupled to the substrate-induced conformation change and resulting removal of the sixth ligand. In contrast, the occurrence of spin state equilibrium in the substrate-bound form can readily be explained by assuming water-ligation in the low-spin form and the change in hydrophobicity of the heme environment by substrate binding (Fig. 12B). This may be additional support for the assumption that the sixth ligand of the low-spin form is a water molecule.

Structural Proposal of the Heme Environment of Cytochrome P-450 and Its Relationship to the Spectral Properties

Based on the discussions in the preceding sections, the following assumption can be made on the heme environment of cytochrome P-450. Cytochrome P-450 may essentially be a penta-coordinated protoheme protein having thiolate as its only internal axial ligand. The heme environment of the cytochrome must be hydrophobic, but the hydrophobicity may not be strong enough to exclude solvent water completely from the heme crevice. In addition, the crevice must have enough space to allow the approach of a water molecule to the heme moiety, because substrates are usually larger than water molecule and the substrate binding site must be in the heme crevice. Thus, a solvent water can bind to the sixth coordination position of the heme iron and the cytochrome may turn into the hexa-coordinated low-spin complex, so-called low-spin cytochrome P-450. It is also likely that the bound water molecule exchanges rapidly with solvent water and that the following equilibrium is established:

$$P\text{-}450 \text{ (high-spin)} + H_2O \rightleftharpoons P\text{-}450\text{-}H_2O \text{ (low-spin)}.$$

Hydrophobicity of the heme environment must affect this equilibrium and may determine the apparent spin state of the cytochrome. The hydrophobicities of the heme environment of various molecular species of cytochrome P-450 may differ. Hydrophobicity must also be altered by binding with a substrate. Furthermore, the equilibrium of the above equation must be affected by temperature. Thus, the reason for molecular species differing in their spin states and of substrate-induced and temperature-dependent spin state changes can uniformly be understood by considering the ligand structure of cytochrome P-450 as above.

REFERENCES

1. Backes, W. L. and Canady, W. J. The interaction of hepatic cytochrome P-450 with organic solvents. The effect of organic solvents on apparent spectral binding constants for hydrocarbon substrates. *J. Biol. Chem.*, **256**, 7213–7227 (1981).

2. Backes, W. L., Hogaboom, M., and Canday, W. J. The true hydrophobicity of microsomal cytochrome P-450 in the rat. Size dependence of the free energy of binding of a series of hydrocarbon substrates from the aqueous phase to the enzyme and to the membrane as derived from spectral binding data. *J. Biol. Chem.*, **257**, 4063–4070 (1982).

3. Chang, C. K. and Dolphin, D. Carbon monoxide binding to pentacoordinate mercaptide-heme complexes: Kinetic study on models for cytochrome P-450. *Proc. Natl. Acad. Sci. U. S.*, **73**, 3338–3342 (1976).

4. Chevion, M., Peisach, J., and Blumberg, W. E. Imidazole, the ligand *trans* to mercaptide in ferric cytochrome P-450. *J. Biol. Chem.*, **252**, 3637–3645 (1977).

5. Cinti, D. L., Sligar, S. G., Gibson, G. G., and Schenkman, J. B. Temperature dependent spin equilibrium of microsomal and solubilized cytochrome P-450 from rat liver. *Biochemistry*, **18**, 36–42 (1979).

6. Cramer, S. P., Dawson, J. H., Hodgson, K. O., and Hagar, L. P. Studies on the ferric form of cytochrome P-450 and chloroperoxidase by extended X-ray absorption fine structure. Characterization of Fe-N and Fe-S distances. *J. Am. Chem. Soc.*, **100**, 7282–7290 (1978).

7. Dawson, J. H., Andersson, L. A., and Sono, M. Spectroscopic interactions of ferric cytochrome P-450$_{cam}$ ligand complexes. Identification of the ligand *trans* to cysteine in the native enzyme. *J. Biol. Chem.*, **257**, 3606–3617 (1982).

8. Dawson, J. H., Holm, R. H., Trudell, J. R., Barth, G., Linder, R. E., Bunnenberg, E., Djerassi, C., and Tang, S. C. Oxidized cytochrome P-450. Magnetic circular dichroism evidence for thiolate ligation in the substrate-bound form. Implications for the catalytic mechanism. *J. Am. Chem. Soc.*, **98**, 3707–3709 (1976).

9. Estabrook, R. W., Coon, M. J., Sato, R., Conney, A. H., Gustafsson, J.-A., Omura, T., and Nebert, D. W. Heralded highlights and harbingers of hope. *In* "Microsomes, Drug Oxidations and Drug Toxicity," ed. R. Sato and R. Kato, pp. 3–11 (1982). Japan Sci. Soc. Press, Tokyo/Wiley-Interscience, New York.

10. Griffin, B. W. and Peterson, J. A. *Pseudomonas putida* cytochrome P-450. The effect of complexes of the ferric hemeprotein of the relaxation of solvent water protons. *J. Biol. Chem.*, **250**, 6445–6451 (1975).

11. Hashimoto, Y., Yamano, T., and Mason, H. S. An electron spin resonance study of microsomal electron transport. *J. Biol. Chem.*, **237**, PC3843–PC3844 (1962).

12. Hashimoto-Yutsudo, C., Imai, Y., and Sato, R. Multiple forms of cytochrome P-450 purified from liver microsomes of phenobarbital- and 3-methylcholanthrene-treated rabbits. II. Spectral properties. *J. Biochem.*, **88**, 505–516 (1980).

13. Haugen, D. A. and Coon, M. J. Properties of electrophoretically homogenous phenobarbital-inducible and β-naphthoflavon-inducible forms of liver microsomal cytochrome P-450. *J. Biol. Chem.*, **251**, 7929–7939 (1976).

14. Ichikawa, Y. and Yamano, T. The role of the hydrophobic bonding in P-450 and the effect of organic compounds on the conversion of P-450 to P-420. *Biochim. Biophys. Acta*, **147**, 518–525 (1967).

15. Iizuka, T. and Yamano, T. Magnetic properties of cytochrome P-450. *In* "Cytochrome P-450," ed. R. Sato and T. Omura, pp. 106–132 (1978). Kodansha, Tokyo/Academic Press, New York.

16. Imai, Y. Interaction of polycyclic hydrocarbons with cytochrome P-450. *In* "Microsomes,

Drug Oxidations, and Drug Toxicity," ed. R. Sato and R. Kato, pp. 53–60 (1982). Japan Sci. Soc. Press, Tokyo/Wiley-Interscience, New York.

17. Imai, Y., Hashimoto-Yutsudo, C., Satake, H., Girardin, A., and Sato, R. Multiple forms of cytochrome P-450 purified from liver microsomes of phenobarbital- and 3-methylcholanthrene-treated rabbits. I. Resolution, purification, and molecular properties. *J. Biochem.*, **88**, 489–503 (1980).

18. Imai, Y. and Sato, R. Conversion of P-450 to P-420 by neutral salts and some other reagents. *Eur. J. Biochem.*, **1**, 419–426 (1967).

19. Imai, Y. and Sato, R. Studies on the substrate interactions with P-450 in drug hydroxylation by liver microsomes. *J. Biochem.*, **62**, 239–249 (1967).

20. Jefcoate, C.R.E. and Gaylor, J. L. Ligand interactions with hemoprotein P-450. II. Influence of phenobarbital and methylcholanthrene induction process on P-450 spectra. *Biochemistry*, **8**, 3464–3472 (1968).

21. Koch, S., Tang, S. C., Holm, R. H., Frankel, R. B., and Ibers, J. A. Ferric porphyrin thiolates. Possible relationship to cytochrome P-450 enzymes and the structure of (*p*-nitrobenzenethiolato) iron (III) protoporphyrin IX dimethyl ester. *J. Am. Chem. Soc.*, **97**, 916–918 (1975).

22. Lange, R., Bonfiles, C., and Debey, P. The low-spin high-spin transition of camphorbound cytochrome P-450. Effects of medium and temperature on equilibrium data. *Eur. J. Biochem.*, **79**, 623–628 (1977).

23. Nemethy, G. Hydrophobic interactions. *Angew. Chem. Int. Edit.*, **6**, 195–280 (1967).

24. Omura, T. and Sato, R. The carbon monoxide-binding pigment of liver microsomes. I. Evidence for its hemoprotein nature. *J. Biol. Chem.*, **239**, 2370–2378 (1964).

25. Omura, T. and Sato, R. The carbon monoxide-binding pigment of liver microsomes. II. Solubilization, purification, and properties. *J. Biol. Chem.*, **239**, 2379–2385 (1964).

26. Ozaki, Y., Kitagawa, T., Kyogoku, Y., Imai, Y., Hashimoto-Yutsudo, C., and Sato, R. Resonance Raman studies of hepatic microsomal cytochrome P-450. Evidence for strong pi basicity of the fifth ligand in the reduced and carbonyl complex forms. *Biochemistry*, **17**, 5826–5831 (1978).

27. Ristau, O., Rein, H., Janig, G.-R., and Ruckpaul, K. Quantitative analysis of the spin equilibrium of cytochrome P-450 LM-2 fraction from rabbit liver microsomes. *Biochim. Biophys. Acta*, **536**, 226–234 (1978).

28. Schenkman, J. B., Remmer, H., and Estabrook, R. W. Spectral studies of drug interaction with hepatic microsomal cytochrome. *Mol. Pharmacol.* **3**, 113–123 (1967).

29. Shimizu, T., Iizuka, T., Shimada, H., Ishimura, Y., Nozawa, T., and Hatano, M. Magnetic circular dichroism studies of cytochrome P-450$_{cam}$. Characterization of axial ligands of ferric and ferrous low-spin complexes. *Biochim. Biophys. Acta*, **670**, 341–354 (1981).

30. Shimizu, T., Nozawa, T., Hatano, M., Imai, Y., and Sato, R. Magnetic circular dichroism studies of hepatic microsomal cytochrome P-450. *Biochemistry*, **14**, 4172–4178 (1975).

31. Stern, J. O. and Peisach, J. A model compound study of the CO-addact of cytochrome P-450. *J. Biol. Chem.*, **249**, 7495–7498 (1974).

32. White, R. E. and Coon, M. J. Heme ligand replacement reactions of cytochrome P-450. Characterization of the bonding atom of the axial ligand *trans* to thiolate as oxygen. *J. Biol. Chem.*, **257**, 3073–3083 (1982).

33. Yoshida, Y., Imai, Y., and Hashimoto-Yutsudo, C. Spectrophotometric examination of exogenous-ligand complexes of ferric cytochrome P-450. Characterization of the axial ligand *trans* to thiolate in the native ferric low-spin form. *J. Biochem.*, **91**, 1651–1659 (1982).

34. Yoshida, Y. and Kumaoka, H. Studies on the substrate-induced spectral change of cytochrome P-450 in liver microsomes. *J. Biochem.*, **78**, 445–468 (1975).
35. Yoshida, Y. Studies on the relationship between the spin-state and the heme environment of ferric cytochrome P-450. *J. Pharm. Dyn.*, **6**, s-89 (1983) (Abstr.).

GANN Monograph on Cancer Research 30, 1985

CHARACTERISTICS OF PURIFIED CYTOCHROME P-450s IN MICROSOMES OF RAT LUNG AND MORRIS HEPATOMA 5123D

Minro Watanabe, Ikuko Sagami, Tetsuo Ohmachi, and Hiroshi Fujii

*Department of Cancer Chemotherapy and Prevention, Research Institute for Tuberculosis and Cancer, Tohoku University**

A major form of pulmonary cytochrome P-450$_{MC}$ (P-450$_{MC}$) was purified approximately 313-fold from lung microsomes in a Buffalo strain of rats treated with 3-methylcholanthrene (MC). The purified preparation contained 12.5 nmol of P-450 per mg protein and the monomeric molecular weight was estimated to be 54,000 daltons by SDS-polyacrylamide gel electrophoresis (SDS-PAGE). The primary structure of pulmonary P-450$_{MC}$ seemingly differed from that of hepatic P-450$_{MC}$, which is a major form of hepatic P-450 from MC-treated rats; the molecular weight of hepatic P-450$_{MC}$ is 56,000 and, different peptide patterns after partial proteolysis with either V8 protease or papain were also observed. In a reconstituted system containing NADPH-cytochrome P-450 reductase and phospholipid, pulmonary P-450$_{MC}$ efficiently catalyzed benzo[a]pyrene (BP) hydroxylation and ethoxycoumarin O-deethylation as hepatic P-450$_{MC}$ did, and in the presence of purified hepatic epoxide hydrolase a higher ratio of 7, 8-diol and of the three unknown fractions and a lower ratio of 3-phenol to the total BP metabolites were estimated in pulmonary P-450$_{MC}$ by high pressure liquid chromatography analysis, when compared to the patterns in hepatic P-450$_{MC}$.

There were at least two forms of P-450, P-450$_{MCI}$ and P-450$_{MCII}$, in microsomes of Morris hepatoma 5123D from MC-treated rats. The electrophoretic mobility of hepatoma P-450$_{MCI}$ and its peptide composition after partial proteolysis with V8 protease were similar to those of hepatic P-450$_{MC}$. The monomeric molecular weight of hepatoma P-450$_{MCII}$ was calculated to be 50,000 daltons on SDS-PAGE. No apparent differences in the spectrophotometric, enzymatic or immunological properties were observed between hepatoma P-450$_{MCI}$ and hepatic P-450$_{MC}$, but in hepatoma P-450$_{MCII}$ the activities of BP hydroxylation, 7-ethoxycoumarin O-deethylation, benzphetamine N-demethylation, and aniline-p-hydroxylation were clearly lower than those in hepatoma P-450$_{MCI}$.

Most of the chemical carcinogens formed in our environment require metabolic activation to exert their deteriorative effects in the target cells. The major activation pathway is an oxidative metabolism, usually catalyzed by the cytochrome P-450 dependent monooxygenase system which has been resolved into at least two catalytic

---

* Seiryo-machi 4-1, Sendai 980, Japan (渡辺民朗, 佐上郁子, 大町鉄雄, 藤井　博).

components, namely, a species of cytochrome P-450 (P-450) and NADPH-cytochrome P-450 reductase (NADPH reductase) and which increases the electrophilicity and reactivity of the parent compounds. Furthermore, multiple forms of P-450 have been isolated and purified from some species of experimental animals. Several forms of liver P-450 were homogeneously purified and extensively characterized in mice (7, 34), rats (14, 29, 40), guinea pigs (2), and rabbits (15, 29).

Chemical carcinogens such as polycyclic aromatic hydrocarbons and nitrosamines, are ubiquitous in the human environment, both in the food and in the atmosphere, and enter the human body through the surface epithelium. The surface area of the respiratory tract is directly exposed to some of these compounds during inhalation. Chemical carcinogens and/or their metabolites can also reach the lung *via* systematic and pulmonary circulation systems (6). Furthermore, it is known that some chemical carcinogens, such as benzo[a]pyrene (BP), 3-methylcholanthrene (MC), and diethyl-nitrosamine, produce lung cancer in mice, rats, and hamsters (27, 35). BP has also been shown to cause *in vitro* malignant transformation of rat tracheal epithelial cells (46).

In lung tissues from experimental animals and humans the metabolism of chemical carcinogens and other xenobiotics has been extensively investigated in both cellular and subcellular preparations, and it was interestingly demonstrated that the charac-teristics of BP hydroxylation differed between lung and liver microsomes from mice (54), guinea pigs (1) and rats (58). It was also reported that between the two tissues certain subtle difference existed in the affinity to NADH for microsomal mixed-function oxidase systems (31) and in the role of the activation of chemical carcinogens for cell-mediated mutagenesis (26).

It is of importance for us to try to purify P-450 from rat lung, and to ascertain whether there is a difference in the properties between the pulmonary P-450 herein reported and hepatic P-450 which has been identified and well characterized.

When compared with normal liver and the host liver from hepatoma bearing rats, many hepatic tumors exhibited significantly lower activity of drug-metabolizing en-zymes, but the decrease of this activity was not related to the growth rate or the grade of differentiation of the tumor tissues (3, 9, 47, 57). After the administration of MC as a potent inducer the apparent induction of such enzymes was observed in certain slower growing tumor lines of Morris hepatoma (9, 47), but not in some lines of rapidly growing hepatoma, *e.g.*, Morris hepatoma 3924-A and Yoshida ascites hepatoma (5).

It is of interest to know whether or not drug metabolizing enzymes of hepatoma are different in their biochemical properties from that of liver from which the hepatoma cell is derived. Watanabe *et al.* (52, 53) previously reported that there were slight dif-ferences in kinetics of microsomal BP hydroxylation between Morris hepatoma 5123D and the host liver from the rat bearing the hepatoma. Further, Miyake *et al.* (33) reported that by means of cyanide titration one and two forms of hemoprotein were detected in the microsomes of rapidly growing tumor line, Morris hepatoma 7777 and slower growing tumor line, 5123C, respectively, whereas rat hepatic hemoprotein exists in at least three spectrally identifiable forms, suggesting the presence of multiple forms of the hemoprotein in hepatomas.

In order to elucidate the biochemical properties of P-450 in the hepatoma cells, we tried to prepare the purified form of P-450 from Morris hepatoma 5123D which is a line of minimal deviation hepatoma (37), and also to learn whether or not the multiple forms of P-450 are present in the hepatoma cells, and finally to ascertain whether or not there are differences in enzymatic, spectrophotometric, and immunological properties of the P-450 between hepatoma and liver which is an original tissue of hepatoma.

Purification of Cytochrome P-450 from Rat Lung

Jernström *et al.* (*23*) first tried to purify P-450 in lung microsomes from MC-treated rats and demonstrated the appearance of BP hydroxylation activity in the reconstituted enzyme system containing a purified P-450 as specific content of 0.66 nmol per mg protein; they also reported that the CO-reduced difference spectrum of the P-450 showed an absorption maxima at 452 nm which is apparently different from the major P-450 in rat liver. It may be necessary to obtain a more highly purified form of pulmonary P-450, because the specific content of that previously reported was still very low compared to the hepatic P-450 usually obtained in our laboratory.

In the experiment herein reported we tried to purify P-450 from rat lung microsomes (*42, 48, 55, 56*). Male Buffalo rats were treated intraperitoneally with MC. The homogenization of lung tissue was performed with an Ultra-Turrax homogenizer (Janke and Kunkel KG, Staufen, F.R.G.) to obtain the microsomal fraction. The results of a typical preparation of pulmonary P-450$_{MC}$, a major P-450 in the microsomal fraction, are outlined in Table I. In the aminooctyl Sepharose chromatography step, P-450 was eluted with the buffer containing 0.08% Emulgen and 0.4% cholate, and no other forms of P-450 were eluted when the Emulgen concentration in the buffer was raised to 0.2%. Masuda-Mikawa *et al.* (*30*) reported that major hepatic P-450s in phenobarbital (PB) or MC-treated rats were eluted with 0.08% Emulgen concentration through aminooctyl Sepharose column, and this was also true in our experimental results. On the contrary, Imai *et al.* (*21*) and Kamataki *et al.* (*24*) mentioned that differentiated requirements of Emulgen concentration as an elution buffer for the purification of P-450 appeared in liver microsomes from PB and MC-treated rabbits and from untreated rats, respectively. The potassium phosphate eluates from the hydroxyapatite column were divided into three fractions, and 80–90% of the total P-450 eluate was recovered in the fraction obtained with 150 mM potassium phosphate buffer as an elution solvent, indicating the presence of P-450$_{MC}$ as a major P-450 in the rat lung. The final fraction expressed 12.5 nmol per mg protein as a specific content approximately 313-fold greater than the content of P-450 in the microsomal

TABLE I. Purification of Pulmonary P-450$_{MC}$ from MC-treated Rats

Fraction	Protein (mg)	Cytochrome P-450			
		Total (nmol)	Specific content (nmol/mg protein)	Yield (%)	Purification (fold)
1. Microsomes	1,334	53.1	0.04	100	1.0
2. Cholate extract	1,202	56.9	0.05	107	1.3
3. Aminooctyl Sepharose eluate	77.5	37.5	0.48	71	12
4. Hydroxyapatite eluate	10.0	19.2	1.92	36	48
5. DEAE-cellulose eluate	1.41	9.35	6.63	18	166
6. CM-Sephadex eluate	0.26	3.26	12.5	6	313

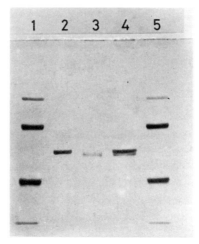

Fig. 1.   SDS-PAGE electrophoresis of purified pulmonary and hepatic P-450$_{MC}$.
Tracks No. 1 and 5 contained standard proteins, tracks No. 2 and 3, hepatic and
pulmonary P-450$_{MC}$, respectively, and track No. 4, both hepatic and pulmonary
P-450$_{MC}$ (*42*).

fraction. The purified sample of the P-450$_{MC}$ was essentially free from NADPH reductase, NADH-cytochrome b_5 reductase, cytochrome b_5, and epoxide hydrolase (EH).
When examined by SDS-polyacrylamide gel electrophoresis (SDS-PAGE), the purified
pulmonary P-450$_{MC}$ gave a single protein band, as shown in Fig. 1. The electrophoretic
mobility of pulmonary P-450$_{MC}$ was significantly different from that of hepatic
P-450$_{MC}$, which is apparently equivalent to either P-450$_c$ (*39*), P-450$_{MC-1}$ (*25*) or P-
450$_{MC-2}$ (*59*). The monomeric molecular weight was estimated to be 54,000 daltons
for the pulmonary P-450$_{MC}$, in contrast to 56,000 for hepatic P-450$_{MC}$.

Characterization of the Pulmonary Cytochrome P-450$_{MC}$

Philpot and Wolf (*36*) reported that from the rabbit lung two P-450s, P-450$_I$ and
P-450$_{II}$, were purified with the specific content of 17–21 and 8–14 nmol per mg protein,
respectively, and that evidence of the identity of P-450$_I$ and rabbit hepatic P-450$_{PB}$
(P-450$_{LM2}$ or form 2) was supported by immunological and enzymatic properties of the
hemoprotein. Liem *et al.* (*28*) and Domin *et al.* (*12*) confirmed the observation of the
induction of a single prominent P-450 by 2,3,7,8-tetrachlorodibenzo-*p*-dioxin (TCDD)
in adult rabbit lung. The similarity of the induced lung P-450 to the hepatic P-450,
form 6, induced by TCDD in newborn rabbit was established by the mobility on
SDS-PAGE, the peptide map of hemoprotein and the specific antigenicity against
each other; such similarity was not established between induced lung P-450 and the
hepatic P-450, form 4, induced by TCDD in adult rabbit. Furthermore, Devereux
et al. (*11*), using immunochemical and cell isolation techniques, showed that the pulmonary P-450$_I$ and P-450$_{II}$ prepared from non-treated rabbits are highly concentrated
in the non-ciliated bronchiolar epithelial (Clara) and alveolar type II cells of the lung.

Table II is summarizes the characteristics of the purified rat pulmonary P-450$_{MC}$
and the purified rat hepatic P-450$_{MC}$. It was clearly observed that there is difference

TABLE II. Comparison of Properties of Purified Major Cytochrome P-450$_{MC}$
in Lung and Liver from Rats Treated with MC

	Lung	Liver
P-450 contents in microsomes (nmol/mg protein)	0.04	1.0
Specific content of purified forms (nmol/mg protein)	12.5	17.0
Purification fold to microsomal P-450	313	17
Minimum molecular weight on SDS-PAGE ($M_r \times 10^{-3}$)	54	56
Peptide composition after partial proteolysis with		
S. aureus V8 protease	Different	
Papain	Different	
α-Chymotrypsin	Similar	
Amino acid composition (mol %)		
Glycine	8.85	7.96
Leucine	11.13	12.05
Other amino acids	Similar	
Maximum of reduced CO-complex (nm)	447.5	447.5
Spin state of heme iron	Low	Low
Catalytic activity in reconstituted system (mol/min/mol P-450)		
BP 3-hydroxylation	11.9	17.1
7-Ethoxycoumarin O-deethylation	23.5	40.0
Benzphetamine N-demethylation	6.3	8.8
Ouchterlony double diffusion with antibody against hepatic P-450$_{MC}$	+	+
	Single fused line	
Inhibitory patterns by antibody against hepatic P-450$_{MC}$		
BP 3-hydroxylation	Completely	Completely
7-Ethoxycoumarin O-deethylation	Completely	Completely

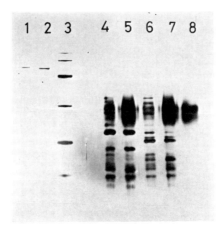

FIG. 2. SDS-PAGE of peptide formed by partial digestion of hepatic and pulmonary P-450$_{MC}$ with *S. aurues* V8 protease. Tracks No. 1 and 2 contained hepatic and pulmonary P-450$_{MC}$ (2.2 μg each), track No. 3 standard protein, tracks No. 4 and 5 hepatic P-450$_{MC}$ (11 μg)+protease (0.5, 2.0 μg), tracks No. 6 and 7 pulmonary P-450$_{MC}$ (11 μg)+protease (0.5, 2.0 μg), and track No. 8, protease alone.

in peptide compositions between pulmonary and hepatic P-450$_{MC}$ after partial proteolysis with proteases such as *Staphylococcus aureus* V8 protease and papain, although α-chymotrypsin gave similar peptide patterns (Fig. 2). Furthermore, the amino acid compositions of pulmonary P-450$_{MC}$ were also different from those of hepatic P-450$_{MC}$, especially in glycine and leucine content, indicating the presence of an unique P-450$_{MC}$ molecule in the rat lung.

In the absorption spectrum of the pulmonary P-450$_{MC}$ from which Emulgen has been removed, the oxidized form has a Soret band at 417 nm and an α and β band at 570 and 535 nm, respectively, indicating a low-spin state of heme iron; the CO-reduced form band is at 447.5 nm, which is similar to a Soret band in the hepatic P-450$_{MC}$.

For the assay of catalytic activity of the pulmonary P-450$_{MC}$ in the reconstituted enzyme system, purified NADPH-reductase was prepared from liver microsomes of MC-treated rat. The activities of BP hydroxylation and 7-ethoxycoumarin deethylation in the pulmonary P-450$_{MC}$ are slightly lower than those in the hepatic P-450$_{MC}$, but apparently higher than those in the hepatic P-450$_{PB}$ which was prepared from liver microsomes of PB-treated rats and which seems equivalent to P-450$_b$ (*40*). In the benzphetamine demethylation, which is a marker oxidation reaction in the reconstituted system containing P-450$_{PB}$, pulmonary P-450$_{MC}$ showed clearly a decreased level in turnover number when compared to the level in hepatic P-450$_{PB}$.

In order to clarify the immunological character of the pulmonary P-450$_{MC}$, its antigenicity was determined using the antibody of rabbit immunoglobulin G (IgG) fraction prepared against the purified hepatic P-450$_{MC}$. In the Ouchterlony double diffusion analysis the antibody reacted well with both pulmonary and hepatic P-450$_{MC}$, and formed a single fused precipitation line without any formation of spur, suggesting immunological identity of the two cytochromes. Furthermore, the antibody clearly inhibited the activities of BP hydroxylation and 7-ethoxycoumarin O-deethylation catalyzed by pulmonary P-450$_{MC}$ as well as by hepatic P-450$_{MC}$ (*18, 51*).

Formation of Benzo[a]pyrene Metabolites with Microsomes and the Reconstituted Enzyme Systems Containing P-450$_{MC}$ from Rat Lung

The major activation pathway of BP metabolism involves the conversion of (−)*trans*-7,8-dihydroxy-7,8-dihydrobenzo[a]pyrene ((−)*t*-7,8-diol) to *r*-7,*t*-8-dihydroxy-*t*-9,10-

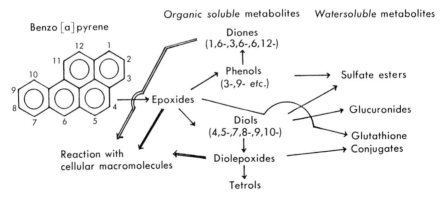

FIG. 3. Benzo[a]pyrene metabolism and the interaction of metabolites to macromolecules (from H. Autrup(*4*)).

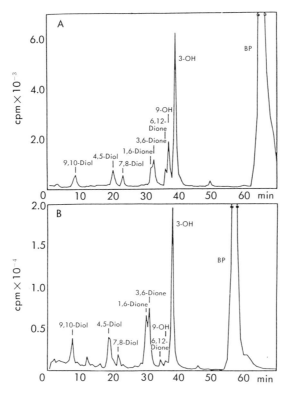

FIG. 4. HPLC patterns of BP metabolites formed *in vitro* by lung microsomes (A) and by reconstituted enzyme systems containing EH (B).

oxy-7,8,9,10-tetrahydrobenzo[a]pyrene ((+)7β,8α-dihydroxy-9α,10α-epoxy-7,8,9,10-tetrahydrobenzo[a]pyrene) (*anti*-diol epoxide) and r-7,t-8-dihydroxy-c-9,10-oxy-7,8,9,10-tetrahydrobenzo[a]pyrene((−)7β,8α-dihydroxy-9β,10β-epoxy-7,8,9,10-tetrahydrobenzo[a]pyrene) (*syn*-diol epoxide) (*49, 62*). The diol epoxides are highly mutagenic and very unstable compounds in aqueous media in which they are quickly hydrolyzed to a pair of tetrahydroxytetrahydrobenzo[a]pyrene (*50, 61*). All BP metabolites were divided into two major groups of compounds, that is, chemicals extracted with organic solvent and with aqueous solution, as shown in Fig. 3. In our experiments the ethylether extracts of the BP metabolites were applied to a TRIROTER high pressure liquid chromatography (HPLC) fitted with a Dupont Zorbax octadecyl trimethoxysilane column (*19, 44*). The HPLC patterns of the BP metabolites from lung microsomes and from the reconstituted enzyme systems containing purified pulmonary P-450$_{MC}$, NADPH-reductase and EH are shown in Fig. 4. Major BP metabolites, that is, three diols (9,10-, 4,5-, and 7,8-), three diones (1,6-, 3,6-, and 6,12-), and two phenols (9- and 3-), were detected in both enzyme systems. In the microsomes 8 major metabolites were clearly separated without any appearance of their unidentified fraction, but in the reconstituted enzyme system the appearance of several unidentified metabolites was confirmed, suggesting some differences of the BP metabolite profile between the microsomes and reconstituted enzyme systems. In general, however, apparent enzyme

TABLE III. Benzo[a]pyrene Metabolites Formed by Liver and Lung Microsomes from MC-treated Rats

Metabolites	Liver (pmol/min/nmol of P-450)	Lung (pmol/min/nmol of P-450)
9,10-Diol	333 (7.9)	234 (6.5)
4,5-Diol	407 (9.7)	264 (7.3)
7,8-Diol	288 (6.9)	146 (4.1)
Σ diols	1,028 (24.5)	644 (17.9)
1,6-Dione 3,6-Dione	835 (19.9)	463 (12.9)
6,12-Dione	125 (3.0)	126 (3.5)
Σ diones	960 (22.9)	589 (16.4)
9-Phenol	607 (14.4)	479 (13.3)
3-Phenol	1,609 (38.3)	1,886 (52.4)
Σ phenols	2,216 (52.7)	2,365 (65.7)
Σ metabolites	4,244 (100)	3,598 (100)

The percentage of each metabolite to total is shown in parentheses.

TABLE IV. Regioselectivity of BP Metabolism by Microsomes in Rat Lung and Liver

Tissue	Strain (sex)	Treatment	Diols 9,10-	4,5-	7,8-	Diones 1,6- 3,6-	6,12-	Phenols 9-	3-	Reporter
Liver	Long-Evans (male)	Control	14[a]	9	10	19	17	6	27	
		MC	20	9	12	23	—	2	25	Holder et al. (19)
		PB	8	12	5	32	—	1	25	
	Sprague-Dawley (male)	Control	5	9	5	31	13	11	28	Hundley et al. (20)
		MC	14	8	12	19	8	13	25	
	WAG (female)	Control	16	8	12	21		8	34	Rouet et al. (38)
	Sprague-Dawley (male)	Control	11	18	9	30		11	21	
		MC	31	12	17	20		8	13	Jefcoate et al. (22)
		PB	6	42	3	42		0	8	
	Buffalo (male)	MC	8	10	7	20	3	14	38	This paper
Lung	Sprague-Dawley (male)	Control	9	9	7	16	8	8	40	Hundley et al. (20)
		MC	5	5	6	12	13	9	37	
	BD VI (female)	Control	4	3	4	55	—	15	20	Sabadie et al. (41)
		PCB[b]	15	4	7	32	—	16	27	
	WAG (female)	Control	8	11	9	15		17	40	Rouet et al. (38)
	Sprague-Dawley (male)	Control	9	18	9	18		15	30	
		MC-I[c]	9	13	6	11		33	28	Jefcoate et al. (22)
		MC-II	9	9	9	13		25	35	
		PB	4	5	11	14		5	60	
	Buffalo (male)	MC	7	7	4	13	4	13	52	This paper

[a] Percentage of each metabolite to total.
[b] PCB, polychlorinated biphenyl.
[c] MC-I, II, assayed after 45 and 90 min incubations with the microsomes, respectively.

reconstitution could be more succesively achieved than the enzyme system in the original lung microsomes.

We tried to compare the HPLC pattern of the BP metabolites between lung and liver microsomes of MC-treated rats. As shown in Table III, the specific activity of the lung was slightly lower than the corresponding liver and lower activities in the formation of the total diols and diones were especially observed. When the specific activity of each metabolite was converted to a percentage of total metabolism, the lung microsomes showed lower levels of 7,8-diol and of a mixture of 1,6- and 3,6- diones in contrast with the higher levels of total phenols (especially 3-phenol) than the liver microsomes. Table IV shows the results of the profile of BP metabolites assayed by different reporters. It was of interest to learn that the detected amounts of diols were lower and the amounts of phenols were higher as BP metabolites in liver microsomes of male Buffalo rats herein reported, as compared to male Long-Evans (19) and male Sprague-Dawley (20, 22) rats treated with MC. In the lung microsomes an apparent increase of 3-phenol formation with a decrease of 6,12-dione formation was also observed in Buffalo rats, compared to the formation of the corresponding metabolites in Sprague-Dawley rats (20, 22). Decreased levels of 7,8-diol and of the 1,6 and 3,6- dione mixture in the lung microsomes were also seen in the Sprague-Dawley and Buffalo rat strains, when compared with the contents in the corresponding liver. Comparing the results with microsomes from corresponding tissues, Autrup et al. (4) stated that the metabolic profile of BP metabolites from rat, mouse, hamster, and human were qualitatively similar in tracheobronchial tissue, and that tetrols and 9,10-diol of BP were predominant metabolites formed by cultured human tissues and hamster trachea, while relatively minor amounts of phenols were formed.

Recently Gozukara et al. (13) reported that different positional and stereoselective oxygenations of BP were observed among the P-450s purified from liver microsomes of MC, β-naphthoflavone (BNF) and PB-induced rats and that the P-450$_{MC}$ and P-450$_{BNF}$ preferred oxidation at the 1,3-, 6-, and 7,8-positions of BP, whereas the P-450$_{PB}$

TABLE V. Benzo[a]pyrene Metabolites by the Reconstituted Monooxygenase System in the Presence and Absence of Purified EH

Metabolites	Hepatic P-450$_{MC}$ EII		Pulmonary P-450$_{MC}$ EH	
	(−) (pmol/min/nmol P-450)	(+)	(−) (pmol/min/nmol P-450)	(+)
Pre-9,10-diol	59 (1.0)	176 (2.7)	213 (2.6)	261 (4.1)
9,10-Diol	301 (4.9)	486 (7.5)	228 (2.8)	514 (8.1)
Unknown I	211 (3.5)	202 (3.1)	371 (4.6)	274 (4.3)
Unknown II	393 (6.5)	76 (1.2)	263 (3.3)	85 (1.3)
4,5-Diol	276 (4.5)	758 (11.7)	369 (4.6)	727 (11.5)
7,8-Diol	115 (1.9)	194 (3.0)	182 (2.3)	226 (3.6)
Unknown III	123 (2.0)	134 (2.1)	242 (3.0)	105 (1.7)
Unknown IV	446 (7.3)	149 (2.3)	331 (4.1)	220 (3.5)
1,6- and 3,6-dione	1,388 (22.8)	1,616 (24.9)	1,706 (21.1)	1,554 (24.5)
6,12-Dione	212 (3.5)	156 (2.4)	164 (2.0)	144 (2.3)
9-Phenol	606 (9.9)	140 (2.2)	804 (9.9)	177 (2.8)
3-Phenol	1,894 (31.1)	2,335 (36.0)	3,145 (38.8)	1,981 (31.3)
Unknown V	73 (1.2)	64 (1.0)	80 (1.0)	69 (1.1)
Total metabolites	6,097 (100)	6,486 (100)	8,098 (100)	6,337 (100)

The percentage of each metabolite to total is shown in parentheses.

TABLE VI. Regioselectivity of BP Metabolism

Tissue	Strain (sex)	Incubation		Pre-9, 10-diol	Diol 9,10-	Unknown		Diols	
		P-450 species	EH/ P-450[a]			I	II	4,5-	7,8-
Liver	Long-Evans (male)	P-450$_c$	0	—	1[b]	—	—	1	1
			24	—	11	—	—	8	11
			72	—	16	—	—	9	12
			240	—	25	—	—	10	12
	Sprague-Dawley (male)	P-450$_{MC}$	0	3	2	1	—	4	8
		P-450$_{BNF}$	0	3	1	1	3	1	4
		P-450$_{PB}$	0	33	10	—	—	9	4
	Sprague-Dawley (male)	P-450$_a$	0	—	23	—	—	6	5
		P-450$_b$	0	—	2	—	—	52	1
		P-450$_e$	0	—	2	—	—	80	—
		P-450$_f$	0	—	21	—	—	45	—
		P-450$_c$	0	—	33	—	—	17	15
		P-450$_d$	0	—	23	—	—	23	8
	Buffalo (male)	P-450$_c$	0	1	5	4	7	5	2
			282	3	8	3	1	12	3
Lung	Buffalo (male)	P-450$_{MC}$	0	3	3	5	3	5	2
			282	4	8	4	1	12	4

[a] Ratio of EH (nmol styrene glycol per min) to P-450 (nmol).

preferred oxidation at the 4,5-position. However, the purified P-450 fractions they used still contained EH, and seemingly remained to be clear in their respective metabolic patterns.

For the reconstituted enzyme system we used NADPH-reductase and EH which were purified from liver of MC-treated rats by the procedures of Yasukochi and Masters (60) and Guengerich et al. (16), respectively. The purified P-450s and NADPH-reductase used contained no detectable EH activity using styrene oxide as a substrate for the enzyme assay. Mutually the purified EH did not contain P-450 species by spectrophotometric analysis. After stopping the reaction by addition of acetone, vitamin E was further added to the incubation mixtures to prevent the spontaneous oxidation of the BP metabolites in our experiments. The patterns of the BP metabolites in the reconstituted enzyme system were carefully compared between pulmonary and hepatic P-450$_{MC}$. As shown in Table V, with the addition of EH into the reconstituted system the specific activity of the total BP metabolites was not changed in the hepatic P-450$_{MC}$, but was slightly decreased in the pulmonary P-450$_{MC}$; an increase of diol formation and a decrease of 9-phenol formation were clearly observed in both the P-450$_{MC}$ The effect of EH on the formation of 3-phenol, however, differed between hepatic and pulmonary P-450$_{MC}$. Under the incubation condition containing purified EH, higher amounts of the pre-9, 10-diol, unknown I and IV fractions and of 7,8-diol, and lower amounts of 3-phenol were detected in pulmonary P-450$_{MC}$ than in hepatic P-450$_{MC}$.

Table VI shows the previously reported results of the HPLC profile of BP metabolites and the effect of EH in the reconstituted enzyme system. Holder et al. (19) reported that in the reconstituted enzyme systems containing hepatic P-450$_{MC}$ purified from Long-Evans strain of immature rats, the formations of diols and 9-phenol were

by the Reconstituted Enzyme System in Rats

Unknown			Diones			Phenols		Reporter
III	IV	V	1,6-	3,6-	6,12-	9-	3-	
—	—	—	32		11	18	28	
—	—	—	32		—	12	19	Holder *et al.* (*19*)
—	—	—	32		—	7	18	
—	—	—	29		—	3	15	
3	2	3	11	12	3	17	29	
3	1	4	10	14	1	17	32	Gozukara *et al.* (*13*)
5	2	11	2	2	2	4	12	
—	—	—	9	11	—	4	44	
—	—	—	6	7	—	3	30	
—	—	—	7	5	—	—	7	Jefcoate *et al.* (*22*)
—	—	—	—	—	—	—	34	
—	—	—	9	12	—	3	13	
—	—	—	11	16	—	5	16	
2	7	—		23	4	10	31	
2	2	—		25	2	2	36	This paper
3	4	—		21	2	10	39	
2	4	—		25	2	3	31	This paper

[b] Percentage of each metabolite to total.

increased and decreased reciprocally after EH addition (Table V), but higher levels of 9,10- and 7,8- diols and a lower level of 3-phenol were relatively determined. It was of interest to note the similar profile of general HPLC patterns of BP metabolites between the results of Gozukara *et al.* (*13*) and our own, but, compared to our reconstituted system containing hepatic P-450$_{MC}$, a high level of 7,8-diol and a low level of 9,10- and 4,5- diols were detected in the hepatic P-450$_{MC}$ system prepared from the Sprague-Dawley strain of rats. It is unclear at the present time whether or not these different BP metabolite ratios observed by different reporters were caused by the various strains of rats used. On the other hand, Jefcoate *et al.* (*22*) reported that even without addition of EH, high levels of the three diol and low levels of phenol were also detected in the system containing hepatic P-450$_c$ from Sprague-Dawley rats.

As mentioned earlier regarding the hepatic tissue, BP is metabolized by lung microsomes and by the reconstituted enzyme systems including pulmonary P-450$_{MC}$ to a wide variety of metabolites including dihydrodiols and phenols of BP. At the present time these studies, however, as reported earlier (*8, 45*), have identified no obvious relationship between BP metabolism by lung tissue and the likely transformation of lung cells to malignant cells.

Purification of Cytochrome P-450 from Morris Hepatoma 5123D

As far as we know, the purification and identification of P-450 in microsomes of hepatoma cells has been performed only by H.W. Strobel and his associates in Houston, and they reported that the purified P-450 in microsomes of Morris hepatoma 5123tc from tumor-bearing rats treated with PB had a specific content of 0.73 nmol per mg protein with purification fold of 9; they confirmed the reconstitution *in vitro* of a drug metabolizing enzyme, which was benzphetamine as a substrate *(43)*. Up to the present time, however, no paper has been offered to our knowledge on the characterized multiple forms of P-450 from the hepatoma cells.

It was confirmed earlier that the induction of BP hydroxylation appeared in microsomes of Morris hepatoma 5123D after the administration of MC *(52, 57)*. Therefore, the hepatoma microsomes were solubilized with sodium cholate in the presence of leupeptin and pepstatin mentioned as protease inhibitors, and at least two forms of P-450, P-450$_{MCI}$ and P-450$_{MCII}$, were obtained *(35a)*. The purification steps of hepatoma P-450$_{MCI}$ are shown in Table VII. P-450$_{MCII}$ was separated from P-450$_{MCI}$ at the step of DEAE-cellulose column chromatography, because the former could be eluted with 40 mM potassium chloride buffer and the latter with 80 mM potassium chloride. The hepatoma P-450$_{MCI}$ was further purified on a CM-Sephadex column, and the final fraction expressed 16.8 nmol per mg protein as a specific content with an approximate 77-fold increase, compared with the content of P-450 in microsomes. The hepatoma P-450$_{MCII}$, on the other hand, expressed 8.25 nmol per mg protein as a specific content

TABLE VII. Purification of Cytochrome P-450$_{MCI}$ in Morris Hepatoma 5123D
of MC-treated Rats

Fractions	Protein (mg)	Cytochrome P-450		Yield (%)	Purification (fold)
		Total content (nmol)	Specific content (nmol/mg protein)		
1. Microsomes	642	136	0.218	100	1.0
2. Cholate extract	282	107	0.379	78.6	1.7
3. Aminooctyl Sepharose eluate	43.5	48.4	1.11	35.6	5.1
4. Hydroxyapatite eluate	7.0	13.1	1.87	9.6	8.6
5. DEAE-cellulose eluate	0.44	6.51	14.9	4.8	68
6. CM-Sephadex eluate	0.15	2.56	16.8	1.9	77

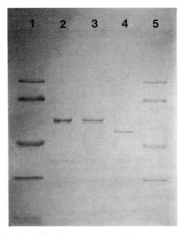

FIG. 5. SDS-PAGE of purified hepatoma P-450$_{MCI}$ and P-450$_{MCII}$ and hepatic P-450$_{MC}$. Tracks No. 1 and 5 contained standard protein, and tracks No. 2, 3, and 4 hepatic P-450$_{MC}$, hepatoma P-450$_{MCI}$, and P-450$_{MCII}$, respectively *(35a)*.

with 1.8% recovery against microsomal P-450. On DEAE-cellulose column the third fraction of P-450 could be eluted, specific content of which was 3.6, and a further purification must thereafter be tried. Each purified P-450, such as $P-450_{MCI}$ and $P-450_{MCII}$, gave nearly an entire major protein band with a minor protein fraction when examined by SDS-PAGE, as shown in Fig. 5. The electrophoretic mobility of the hepatoma $P-450_{MCI}$ was similar to that of hepatic $P-450_{MC}$ ($P-450_c$), estimated to be 56,000 daltons in monomeric molecular weight, and even after the partial proteolysis with V8 protease a clear similarity in the peptide composition was observed between hepatoma $P-450_{MCI}$ and hepatic $P-450_{MC}$. On the other hand, the mobility of hepatoma $P-450_{MCII}$ on SDS-PAGE was significantly different from that of hepatoma $P-450_{MCI}$, and the molecular weight of $P-450_{MCII}$ was calculated to be 50,000 daltons.

Characterization of Hepatoma Cytochrome P-450s

Table VIII shows the properties of the purified hepatoma $P-450_{MCI}$ and $P-450_{MCII}$ in tumor-bearing rats treated with MC, compared to those of hepatic $P-450_{MC}$. By spectrophotometric analysis Soret bands of reduced CO-complex in the hepatomas $P-450_{MCI}$ and $P-450_{MCII}$ were 446.5 and 451 nm, respectively, and the peak value of the $P-450_{MCI}$ seemed similar to that of hepatic $P-450_{MC}$. On the other hand, no difference in the spin state of heme iron was observed between $P-450_{MCI}$ and $P-450_{MCII}$, because in the absorption spectrum after removal of Emulgen the oxidized form of each hepatoma P-450 had a Soret band at 417 nm.

The assay of catalytic activity was performed in the reconstituted enzyme system

TABLE VIII.   Comparison of Properties of Major P-450s in Hepatoma 5123D and Liver from MC-treated Rats

	Hepatoma 5123D		Rat liver
	$P-450_{MCI}$	$P-450_{MCII}$	$P-450_{MC}$
P-450 content in microsomes (nmol/mg protein)	0.22		1.0
Specific content of purified forms (nmol/mg protein)	16.8	8.25	20.0
Purification fold to microsomal P-450	76	38	20
Molecular weight on SDS-PAGE ($M_r \times 10^3$)	56	50	56
Maximum of reduced CO-complex (nm)	446.5	451	447
Spin state of heme iron	Low	Low	Low
Catalytic activities in reconstituted system (nmol/min/nmol P-450)			
BP 3-hydroxylation	19.2	0.50	23.7
7-Ethoxycoumarin O-deethylation	34.6	ND	53.4
Benzphetamine N-demethylation[a]	2.66	0.66	2.93
Benzphetamine N-demethylation[b]	0.77	0.34	0.76
Aniline p-hydroxylation	1.65	0.44	1.04
Aminopyrin N-demethylation	2.47	ND	0.42
p-Nitroanisole O-demethylation	2.15	0.39	1.68
Antigenicity in Ouchterlony double diffusion analysis			
Towards antibody hepatic $P-450_{MC}$	+	−	+

[a] NADPH oxidation.

[b] Formaldehyde formation.

ND, not detectable.

containing purified hepatoma P-450 and hepatoma NADPH-reductase. The NADPH-reductase used was purified from hepatoma microsomes in MC-treated rats. After elution of P-450 with a buffer solution containing 0.08% Emulgen 913 by ω-amino-n-octyl Sepharose 4B, a solution containing 0.15% sodium cholate and 0.35% sodium deoxycholate was used as an elution buffer to obtain a fraction of NADPH-reductase. Further purification of NADPH-reductase was performed according to Yasukochi and Masters (60), and the specific activity in the final fraction was 45 units per mg protein. The turnover numbers of BP hydroxylation and 7-ethoxycoumarin O-de-ethylation in hepatoma P-450$_{MCI}$ were 19.2 and 34.6 nmol per min per mg protein, respectively, apparently higher than those in hepatoma P-450$_{MCII}$. However, the enzyme activities of benzphetamine and aminopyrine N-demethylation, aniline p-hydroxylation, and p-nitroanisole O-demethylation in hepatoma P-450$_{MCI}$ were clearly low, indicating that hepatoma P-450$_{MCI}$ is similar in catalytic properties to hepatic P-450$_{MC}$. In hepatoma P-450$_{MCII}$ the activities of drug metabolizing enzymes assayed were low compared with hepatoma P-450$_{MCI}$, suggesting the presence of multiple form of P-450 in hepatoma microsomes.

In order to examine the immunological identities of hepatoma P-450$_{MCI}$ and hepatic P-450$_{MC}$, an antibody against the latter was prepared from rabbit serum. In Ouchterlony double diffusion analysis hepatoma P-450$_{MCI}$ reacted well to the antibody against hepatic P-450$_{MC}$ with a single fused line but hepatoma P-450$_{MCII}$ did not, indicating an apparent difference in immunological property between these two hepatoma P-450s.

In summary, multiple forms of P-450 were observed in microsomes of Morris hepatoma 5123D and a profile of DEAE-cellulose column chromatography showed it to be at least three forms of P-450 species, P-450$_{MCI}$, P-450$_{MCII}$, and the other P-450 in a ratio of 2:1:1. Experiments are being done now to determine whether a P-450$_{MCII}$ hepatoma is present in hepatoma from non-treated tumor-bearing rats and also in liver from non-treated and MC-treated tumor-bearing rats.

When considering the mechanism of induction of BP metabolizing enzyme in mouse hepatoma, two variant cells that were defective in the cytosolic receptor and in translocation of the inducer-receptor complex to the nucleus, respectively, were reported (17, 32). It is important to clarify which hepatoma P-450 reacts well with each xenobiotic in relation to chemical carcinogenesis and to the effectiveness of cancer chemotherapeutica.

Acknowledgments

We wish to express our hearty gratitude to Mr. K. Kikuchi and Miss M. Hirata for their help in performing these experiments and in preparation of the manuscript. This work was supported in part by a Grant-in-Aid for Cancer Research from the Ministry of Education, Science and Culture, Japan and by a grant from the Japan Tobacco and Salt Public Corporation. BP metabolites were received from the NCI Chemical Carcinogen Reference Standard Repository, a function of the Division of Cancer Cause and Prevention, NCI, NIH, Bethesda, U.S.A.

REFERENCES

1. Abe, T. and Watanabe, M. Genetic differences in the induction of aryl hydrocarbon hydroxylase and its components by 3-methylcholanthrene in liver and lung microsomes among four strains of guinea pigs. *Biochem. Pharmacol.*, **31**, 2077–2082 (1982).

2. Abe, T. and Watanabe, M. Purification and characterization of three forms of microsomal cytochrome P-450 in liver from 3-methylcholanthrene-treated guinea pigs. *Mol. Pharmacol.*, **23**, 258–264 (1983).

3. Adamson, R. H. and Fouts, J. R. The metabolism of drugs by hepatic tumors. *Cancer Res.*, **21**, 667–672 (1961).

4. Autrup, H., Graftstrom, R. C., and Harris, C. C. Metabolism of chemical carcinogens by tracheobronchial tissues. *In* "Organ and Species Specificity in Chemical Carcinogenesis," ed. R. Langenbach, S. Nesnow, and J. M. Rice, pp. 473–494 (1983). Plenum Publishing, New York.

5. Barone, C., Gentiloni, N., Bartoloni, C., Gambassi, G., and Terranova, T. Effects of phenobarbital and 3-methylcholanthrene treatment on microsomes of Morris hepatoma 3924-A, tumor-bearing and normal rat liver. *Oncology*, **36**, 1–6 (1979).

6. Boyd, M. R. Biochemical mechanisms in chemical-induced lung injury: roles of metabolic activation. *CRC Crit. Rev. Toxicol.*, 103–176 (1980).

7. Chen, Y.-T., Lang, M. A., Jensen, N. M., Negishi, M., Tukey, R. H., Sidransky, E., Guenther, T. M., and Nebert, D. W. Similarities between mouse and rat-liver microsomal cytochromes P-450 induced by 3-methylcholanthrene. *Eur. J. Biochem.*, **122**, 361–368 (1982).

8. Cohen, G. M. and Moore, B. P. Metabolism of benzo[a]pyrene and its major metabolites by respiratory tissues. *In* "Carcinogenesis," ed. P. W. Jones and R. I. Freudenthal, Vol. 3, pp. 325–339 (1978). Raven Press, New York.

9. Conney, A. H. and Burns, J. J. Induced synthesis of oxidative enzymes in liver microsomes by polycyclic hydrocarbons and drugs. *Adv. Enzyme Regul.*, **1**, 189–214 (1963).

10. Deutsch, J., Lantz, J. C., Yang, S. K., Gelboin, H. V., Chiang, Y. L., Vatsis, K. P., and Coon, M. J. Regio- and stereoselectivity of various forms of purified cytochrome P-450 in the metabolism of benzo[a]pyrene and (-)*trans*-7,8-dihydroxy-7,8-dihydrobenzo[a]pyrene as shown by product formation and binding to DNA. *Proc. Natl. Acad. Sci. U. S.*, **75**, 3123–3127 (1978).

11. Devereux, T. R., Serabjit-Singh, C. J., Slaughter, S. R., Wolf, C. R., Philpot, R. M., and Fouts, J. R. Identification of cytochrome P-450 isozymes in non-ciliated bronchiolar epithelial (Clara) and alveolar type II cells isolated from rabbit lung. *Exp. Lung Res.*, **2**, 221–230 (1981).

12. Domin, B. A., Philpot, R. M., Warren, B. L., and Serabjit-Singh, C. J. Modulation of the levels of cytochrome P-450 isozymes in rabbit lung. *In* "Extrahepatic Drug Metabolism and Chemical Carcinogenesis," ed. J. Rydström, J. Montelius, and M. Bengtsson, pp. 43–49 (1983). Elsevier Biomedical, Amsterdam.

13. Gozukara, E. M., Guengerich, F. P., Miller, H., and Gelboin, H. V. Different patterns of benzo[a]pyrene metabolism of purified cytochrome P-450 from methylcholanthrene, β-naphthoflavone and phenobarbital treated rats. *Carcinogenesis*, **3**, 129–133 (1982).

14. Guengerich, F. P., Dannan, G. A., Wright, S. T., Martin, M. V., and Kaminsky, L. S. Purification and characterization of liver microsomal cytochromes P-450: Electrophoretic, spectral, catalytic, and immunochemical properties and inducibility of eight isozymes isolated from rats treated with phenobarbital or β-naphthoflavone. *Biochemistry*, **21**, 6019–6030 (1982).

15. Guengerich, F. P., Wang, P., and Davidson, N. K., Estimation of isozymes of microsomal cytochrome P-450 in rats, rabbits, and humans using immunochemical staining coupled with sodium dodecyl sulfate-polyacrylamide gel electrophoresis. *Biochemistry*, **21**, 1698–1706 (1982).

16. Guengerich, F. P., Wang, P., Mitchell, M. B., and Mason, P. S. Rat and human liver microsomal epoxide hydratase. Purification and evidence for the existance of multiple forms. *J. Biol. Chem.*, **254**, 12248–12254 (1979).

17. Hankinson, O. Evidence that benzo[a]pyrene-resistant, aryl hydrocarbon hydroxylase-deficient variants of mouse hepatoma line, Hepa-1, are mutational in origin. *Somat. Cell Genet.*, **7**, 373–388 (1981).

18. Harada, N. and Omura, T. Selective induction of two different molecular species of cytochrome P-450 by phenobarbital and 3-methylcholanthrene. *J. Biochem.*, **89**, 237–248 (1981).

19. Holder, G., Yagi, H., Dansette, P., Jerina, D. M., Levin, W., Lu, A.Y.H., and Conney, A. H. Effects of inducers and epoxide hydrolase on the metabolism of benzo[a]pyrene by liver microsomes and a reconstituted system: Analysis by high pressure liquid chromatography. *Proc. Natl. Acad. Sci. U. S.*, **71**, 4356–4360 (1974).

20. Hundley, S. G. and Freudenthal, R. I. A comparison of benzo[a]pyrene metabolism by liver and lung microsomal enzymes from 3-methylcholanthrene treated rhesus monkeys and rats. *Cancer Res.*, **37**, 3120–3125 (1977).

21. Imai, Y., Hashimoto-Yutsudo, C., Satake, H., Girardin, A., and Sato, R. Multiple forms of cytochrome P-450 purified from liver microsomes of phenobarbital- and 3-methylcholanthrene-pretreated rabbits. I. Resolution, purification, and molecular properties. *J. Biochem.*, **88**, 489–503 (1980).

22. Jefcoate, C. R., Christou, M., Keller, G. M., Turner, C. R., and Wilson, N. M. A kinetic approach to polycyclic hydrocarbon activation. *In* "Extrahepatic Drug Metabolism and Chemical Carcinogenesis," ed. J. Rydström, J. Montelius, and M. Bengtsson, pp. 449–458 (1983). Elsevier Science, Amsterdam.

23. Jernström, B., Capdevila, J., Jakobsson, S., and Orrenius, S. Solubilization and partial purification of cytochrome P-450 from rat lung microsomes. *Biochem. Biophys. Res. Commun.*, **64**, 814–822 (1975).

24. Kamataki, J., Maeda, K., Yamazoe, Y., Nagai, T., and Kato, R. Partial purification and characterization of cytochrome P-450 responsible for the occurrence of sex difference in drug metabolism in the rat. *Biochem. Biophys. Res. Commun.*, **103**, 1–7 (1981).

25. Kuwahara, S., Harada, N., Omura, T., and Mannering, G. J. Purification of five forms of cytochrome P-450 from rat liver microsomes and their contributions to microsomal drug oxidations. *In* "Microsomes, Drug Oxidations and Drug Toxicity," ed. R. Sato and R. Kato, pp. 79–80 (1982). Japan Sci. Soc. Press, Tokyo / Wiley-Interscience, New York.

26. Langenbach, R., Nesnow, S., Tompa, A., Gingell, R., and Kuszynski, C. Lung and liver cell-mediated mutagenesis systems: Specificities in the activation of chemical carcinogens. *Carcinogenesis*, **2**, 851–858 (1981).

27. Laskin, S. and Sellakumar, A. Models in chemical respiratory carcinogenesis. *In* "Experimental Lung Cancer," ed. E. Karbe and J. F. Park, pp. 7–19 (1974). Springer-Verlag, New York.

28. Liem, H. H., Muller-Eberhard, U., and Johnson, E. F. Differential induction by 2, 3, 7, 8-tetrachlorodibenzo-*p*-dioxin of multiple forms of rabbit microsomal cytochrome P-450: Evidence for tissue specificity. *Mol. Pharmacol.*, **18**, 565–570 (1980).

29. Lu, A.Y.H. and West, S. B. Multiplicity of mammalian microsomal cytochromes P-450. *Pharmacol. Rev.*, **31**, 277–295 (1980).

30. Masuda-Mikawa, R., Fujii-Kuriyama, Y., Negishi, M., and Tashiro, U. Purification

and partial characterization of hepatic microsomal cytochrome P-450s from phenobarbital- and 3-methylcholanthrene-treated rats. *J. Biochem.*, **86**, 1383–1394 (1979).

31. Matsubara, T., Prough, R. A., Burke, M. D., and Estabrook, R. W. The preparation of microsomal fraction of rodent respiratory tract and their characterization. *Cancer Res.*, **34**, 2196–2203 (1974).

32. Miller, A. G., Israel, D., and Whitlock, J. P., Jr. Biochemical and genetic analysis of variant mouse hepatoma cells defective in the induction of benzo[a]pyrene-metabolizing enzyme activity. *J. Biol. Chem.*, **258**, 3523–3527 (1983).

33. Miyake, Y., Gaylor, J. L., and Morris, H. P. Abnormal microsomal cytochromes and electron transport in Morris hepatomas. *J. Biol. Chem.*, **249**, 1980–1987 (1974).

34. Nebert, D. W. and Negishi, M. Multiple forms of cytochrome P-450 and the importance of molecular biology and evolution. *Biochem. Pharmacol.*, **31**, 2311–2317 (1982).

35. Nettesheim, P. and Griesemer, R. A. Experimental models for studies of respiratory tract carcinogenesis. *In* "Pathogenesis and Therapy of Lung Cancer," ed. C. C. Harris, pp. 75–188 (1978). Marcel Dekker, New York.

35a. Ohmachi, T., Sagami, I., Fujii, H., and Watanabe, M. Microsomal monooxygenase system in Morris hepatoma: Purification and characterization of cytochromes P-450 from Morris hepatoma 5123D of 3-methylcholanthrene-treated rats. *Arch. Biochem. Biophys.*, **235**, in press (1984).

36. Philpot, R. M. and Wolf, C. R. The properties and distribution of the enzymes of pulmonary cytochrome P-450-dependent monooxygenase systems. *Rev. Biochem. Toxicol.*, **3**, 51–76 (1981).

37. Potter, V. R., Watanabe, M., Pitot, H. C., and Morris, H. P. Systematic oscillations in metabolic activity in rat liver and hepatomas. Survey of normal diploid and other hepatoma lines. *Cancer. Res.*, **29**, 55–78 (1969).

38. Rouet, P., Alexandrov, K., Markovits, P., Frayssinet, C., and Dansette, P. M. Metabolism of benzo[a]pyrene by brain microsomes of fetal and adult rats and mice. Induction by 5,6-benzoflavone, comparison with liver and lung microsomal activities. *Carcinogenesis*, **2**, 919–926 (1981).

39. Ryan, D. E., Thomas, P. E., Korzeniowski, D., and Levin, W. Separation and characterization of highly purified forms of liver microsomal cytochrome P-450 from rats treated with polychlorinated biphenyls, phenobarbital, and 3-methylcholanthrene. *J. Biol. Chem.*, **254**, 1365–1374 (1979).

40. Ryan, D. E., Thomas, P. E., Reik, L. M., and Levin, W. Purification, characterization and regulation of five rat hepatic microsomal cytochrome P-450 isozymes. *Xenobiotica*, **12**, 727–744 (1982).

41. Sabadie, N., Richter-Reichhelm, H. B., Saracci, R., Mohr, V., and Bartsch, H. Interindividual differences in oxidative benzo[a]pyrene metabolism by normal and tumorous surgical lung specimens from 105 lung cancer patients. *Int. J. Cancer*, **27**, 417–425 (1981).

42. Sagami, I. and Watanabe, M. Purification and characterization of pulmonary cytochrome P-450 from 3-methylcholanthrene-treated rats. *J. Biochem.*, **93**, 1499–1508 (1983).

43. Saine, S. E. and Strobel, H. W. Drug metabolism in liver tumors. Resolution of components and reconstitution of activity. *Mol. Pharmacol.*, **12**, 649–657 (1976).

44. Selkirk, J. K., Croy, R. G., Roller, P. P., and Gelboin, H. V. High-pressure liquid chromatographic analysis of benzo[a]pyrene metabolism and covalent binding and the mechanism of action of 7, 8-benzoflavone and 1, 2-epoxy-3, 3, 3-trichloropropane. *Cancer Res.*, **23**, 3474–3480 (1974).

45. Smith, B. R. and Bend, J. R. Metabolic interactions of hydrocarbons with mammalian lung. *Rev. Biochem. Toxicol.*, **3**, 77–122 (1981).

46. Steele, V. E., Marchok, A. C., and Cohen, G. M. Transformation of rat tracheal epithe-

lial cells of benzo[a]pyrene and its metabolites. *Cancer Lett.*, **8**, 291–298 (1980).

47. Sugimura, T., Ikeda, K., Hirota, K., Hozumi, M., and Morris, H. P. Chemical, enzymatic, and cytochrome assays of microsomal fraction of hepatomas with different growth rates. *Cancer Res.*, **26**, 1711–1716 (1966).

48. Tamura, Y., Abe, T., and Watanabe, M. Partial purification of pulmonary cytochrome P-448 from 3-methylcholanthrene-treated rats. *J. Toxicol. Sci.*, **6**, 71–81 (1981).

49. Thakker, D. R., Yagi, H., Akagi, H., Koreeda, M., Lu, A.Y.H., Levin, W., Wood, A. W., Conney, A. H., and Jerina, D. M. Metabolism of benzo[a]pyrene. Vl Stereoselective metabolism of benzo[a]pyrene and benzo[a]pyrene 7,8-dihydrodiol to diol epoxides. *Chem.-Biol. Interact.*, **16**, 281–300 (1977).

50. Thakker, D. R., Yagi, H., Lu, A.Y.H., Levin, W., Conney, A. H., and Jerina, D. M. Metabolism of benzo[a]pyrene. IV Conversion of (±)*trans*-7, 8-dihydroxy-7, 8-dihydrobenzo[a]pyrene to the highly mutagenic 7, 8-diol-9, 10-epoxides. *Proc. Natl. Acad. Sci. U. S.*, **73**, 3381–3385 (1976).

51. Thomas, P. E., Korzeniowski, P., Ryan, D., and Levin, W. Preparation of monospecific antibodies against two forms of rat liver cytochrome P-450 and quantitation of these antigens in microsomes. *Arch. Biochem. Biophys.*, **192**, 524–532 (1979).

52. Watanabe, M., Konno, K., and Sato, H. Aryl hydrocarbon hydroxylase in Morris hepatoma 5123D. *Gann*, **66**, 499–503 (1975).

53. Watanabe, M., Konno, K., and Sato, H. Properties of aryl hydrocarbon hydroxylase in microsomes of Morris hepatoma 5123D and the host liver. *Gann*, **66**, 505–511 (1975).

54. Watanabe, M., Konno, K., and Sato, H. Properties of aryl hydrocarbon (benzo[a]pyrene) hydroxylase in lung microsomes of mice. *Gann*, **69**, 1–8 (1978).

55. Watanabe, M., Sagami, I., Abe, T., and Ohmachi, T. Purification and properties of cytochrome P-450$_{MC}$ from rat lung microsomes and its role to activation of chemical carcinogens. *In* "Cytochrome P-450. Biochemistry, Biophysics and Environmental Implications," ed. E. Hietanen, M. Laitinen, and O. Hänninen, pp. 649–652 (1982). Elsevier Biomedical, Amsterdam.

56. Watanabe, M., Sagami, I., and Ohmachi, T. Characterization of purified cytochrome P-450 in the rat lung. *In* "Extrahepatic Drug Metabolism and Chemical Carcinogenesis," ed. J. Rydström, J. Montelius, and M. Bengtsson, pp. 51–55 (1983). Elsevier Science, Amsterdam.

57. Watanabe, M., Potter, V. R., and Morris, H. P. Benzpyrene hydroxylase activity and its induction by methylcholanthrene in Morris hepatomas, in host livers, in adult livers, and in rat liver during development. *Cancer Res.*, **30**, 263–273 (1970).

58. Wiebel, F. J., Leutz, J. C., Diamond, L., and Gelboin, H. V. Aryl hydrocarbon (benzo[a]pyrene) hydroxylase in microsomes from rat tissues: Differential inhibition and stimulation by benzoflavones and organic solvents. *Arch. Biochem. Biophys.*, **144**, 78–86 (1971).

59. Wolf, C. R. and Oesch, F. Isolation of a high spin form of cytochrome P-450 induced in rat liver by 3-methylcholanthrene. *Biochem. Biophys. Res. Commun.*, **111**, 504–511 (1983).

60. Yasukochi, Y. and Masters, B.S.S. Some properties of a detergent-solubilized NADPH-cytochrome *c* reductase purified by biospecific affinity chromatography. *J. Biol. Chem.*, **251**, 5337–5344 (1976).

61. Yang, S. K., McCourt, D. W., and Gelboin, H. V. The mechanism of hydrolysis of the non-K-region benzo[a]pyrene diol epoxide *r*-7, *t*-8-dihydroxy-*t*-9, 10-oxy-7, 8, 9, 10-tetrahydrobenzo[a]pyrene. *J. Am. Chem. Soc.*, **99**, 5130–5134 (1977).

62. Yang, S. K., McCourt, D. W., Leutz, J. C., and Gelboin, H. V. Benzo[a]pyrene diol epoxides: mechanism of enzymatic formation and optically active intermediates. *Science*, **196**, 1199–1201 (1977).

LOCALIZATION OF CYTOCHROME P-450 IN RAT LIVER NUCLEI: ITS POSSIBLE SIGNIFICANCE IN THE CHEMICAL CARCINOGENESIS

Yutaka Tashiro, Shiro Matsuura, and Koichiro Omori

*Department of Physiology, Kansai Medical University**

Localization of cytochrome P-450 in rat liver nuclei was investigated by quantitative ferritin immunoelectron microscopy using mono-specific antibodies against the major molecular species of 3-methyl-cholanthrene- and phenobarbital-induced cytochrome P-450. Ferritin particles were formed to exist exclusively on the cytoplasmic surface of the outer nuclear envelopes, and neither the nucleoplasmic surface of the inner membrane nor the cisternal surface of either the outer or inner membrane of the envelopes showed any labeling with ferritin.

These results indicate that a marked heterogeneity exists in the enzyme distribution between the outer and inner membranes of the nuclear envelope. Ferritin particles were present on the outer membrane up to the outer annuli of the pore complexes, suggesting that the nuclear pore complexes function as a diffusion barrier of cytochrome P-450 molecules between the two membranes.

Nuclear envelope-endoplasmic reticulum (ER) relationships were investigated by observing a number of nuclei prefixed by perfusion with dilute glutaraldehyde. These nuclei sometimes were associated with rough ER, and occasional continuity of the outer nuclear membrane with rough ER membrane was observed.

When unfixed nuclei were incubated with the conjugates, we occasionally found small vesicles heavily labeled with ferritin particles within the nuclear matrix. These inclusion bodies were probably formed by the internalization of either the nuclear envelopes or ER membranes. We cannot, however, deny the possibility that such inclusion bodies may also have been formed *in vivo*. It was suggested that the existence of cytochrome P-450 in the invaginated nuclear envelopes or in the nuclear inclusion bodies is significant in the process of chemical carcinogenesis.

The covalent binding of carcinogenic polycyclic aromatic hydrocarbons to DNA usually requires an initial metabolism of the compound by a mixed function oxidation system including cytochrome P-450 (*11, 23*). The instability of carcinogenic polycyclic aromatic hydrocarbons implies that proximity of the site of generation of these metabolites to the site of DNA modification may be significant in determining the extent of the DNA alteration.

For many years, cytochrome P-450 was considered exclusively a microsomal en-

---

* Fumizonocho 1, Moriguchi, Osaka 570, Japan (田代　裕, 松浦志郎, 大森浩一郎).

zyme. If true, ultimate carcinogenic metabolites would be required to travel a long distance from the endoplasmic reticulum (ER) to the nucleoplasm and the possibility of these highly reactive ultimate carcinogens successfully gaining access to the nuclear DNA under these circumstances appeared small.

Recently, however, biochemical evidence has been presented that cytochrome P-450 is not limited to the ER but is present in nuclear envelopes and even in the nuclear interior (3, 16, 23–25, 28). Biochemical evidence for the involvement of the nuclear envelopes in the activation of procarcinogens was also presented (15). Since the mass of nuclear envelope in the cell is approximately 1% of the total mass of microsomal membrane proteins (3, 6), the possibility exists that cytochrome P-450 is not associated with nuclei but with the contaminating ER membranes.

We recently developed a quantitative immunoelectron microscopic technique and applied it successfully to the analysis of intracellular distribution of cytochrome P-450 molecules in rat liver (19, 20). Using this technique, we can easily determine the distribution of cytochrome P-450 on the membranous organelles without purifying them. We asked whether or not cytochrome P-450 molecules exist in the nuclear envelope. If yes, we sought to learn where and how they exist, either homogeneously on both the outer and inner membrane of the envelopes or exclusively on one of them. We asked too whether or not they also exist within the nuclear interior.

Details of the quantitative immunoelectron microscopic techniques for the intracellular distribution of cytochrome P-450 molecules have been described in detail elsewhere (19, 20). Briefly, the major form of cytochrome P-450 in hepatic microsomes from phenobarbital (PB)-treated rats (P-450 (PB)) or in those from 3-methylcholanthrene (MC)-treated rats (P-450 (MC)) was purified (18). Antisera against the purified P-450(PB) and P-450(MC) were elicited in rabbits and the antibodies were prepared by ammonium sulfate fractionation followed by DEAE-cellulose chromatography.

Cytochrome P-450 was also partially purified from rat liver nuclei. Ouchterlony double diffusion analysis indicated that the nuclear P-450 is immunologically indistinguishable from its microsomal counterpart, as reported by Thomas et al. (27). We therefore used the antibodies against microsomal cytochrome P-450(PB) and P-450(MC) in the present experiment. The antibodies were coupled to ferritin using glutaraldehyde and the ferritin-anti P-450(PB) and P-450(MC) antibody conjugates with a molar ratio of immunoglobulin G (IgG) to ferritin of ~1: 1 were isolated as described previously (19). Nuclei or nuclear envelopes were incubated with ferritin antibody conjugates at the saturation level, and the number of ferritin particles per μm of the envelope membranes was calculated. In this article the results of the previous papers reported from this laboratory (21, 22) will be summarized and discussed more in detail.

Biochemical Studies of Distribution and Induction of Cytochrome P-450 in the Nuclear Envelopes

Table I shows the cytochrome P-450 content and the metabolic activities of the liver nuclear envelopes that were isolated from control, MC-, and PB-treated rats. PB treatment failed to increase either the cytochrome P-450 content or the enzyme activity in the nuclear envelope preparations while treatment with MC markedly increased the content and the metabolic activities of benzo[a]pyrene hydroxylase and

TABLE I. Cytochrome P-450s Content and Metabolic Activities[a] in Control
and Treated Rats[b]

Treatment	P-450 content (nmol/mg P[c])	Turnover number		
		Benzo[a]pyrene	Benzphetamine	7-Ethoxycoumarin
		(nmol product formed/nmol P-450/min)		
Control	1.75	2.63	3.2	1.02
MC	4.25	8.46	4.0	8.18
PB	1.47	1.90	3.8	1.04

[a] Turnover numbers.
[b] Mean of two preparations of nuclear envelopes.
[c] Phospholipid-P.

7-ethoxycoumarine O-deethylase. This result is essentially in agreement with the biochemical results of Kasper *et al.* (*6, 13, 14*), Rogan *et al.* (*24*), and Sagara *et al.* (*26*).

Distribution of Cytochrome P-450 on the Various Surfaces of the Nuclear Envelopes

Photo 1 shows rat liver nuclei from control (A), PB- (B), and MC- (C) treated rats incubated with anti P-450(MC) antibody conjugates. It is evident that the number of ferritin particles bound to the envelopes increased markedly when anti P-450(MC) antibody conjugates were incubated with the nuclei from MC-treated rat liver. Essentially similar results were obtained when anti P-450(PB) antibody conjugates were incubated with the nuclei from PB-treated rat liver (data not shown). Results of the quantitative analyses are shown in Table II. In agreement with Kasper *et al.* (*6, 14*), cytochrome P-450(MC) increased markedly in the nuclear envelope from MC-treated rat liver (3.8×). This result is interesting because P-450(MC) is mainly responsible for the activation of benzo[a]pyrene (*9*), which is an ubiquitous environmental pollutant that may cause cancer in humans.

A slight increase in the ferritin particles was also observed when anti P-450(PB) antibody conjugates were incubated with the nuclei from PB-treated rat liver (1.5×). The fact that the total amount of cytochrome P-450 in the nuclear envelope did not

TABLE II. Binding of Ferritin-antibody Conjugates to the Outer Nuclear
Membranes in Control and Treated Rats

Source of hepatic nuclei	Incubated antibody conjugates	Number of ferritin particles bound per μm of nuclear envelopes[a]
Control	Anti-PB-P-450 antibody	38.7 (100%)
PB-treated	Anti-PB-P-450 antibody	56.7 (150%)
MC-treated	Anti-PB-P-450 antibody	27.0 (68%)
Control	Anti-MC-P-450 antibody	17.1 (100%)
PB-treated	Anti-MC-P-450 antibody	17.2 (101%)
MC-treated	Anti-MC-P-450 antibody	57.6 (381%)
MC-treated	Control IgG	2.7

[a] Average of two morphometrical analyses. Ferritin particles counted were 500–1,000 for each measurement, and the total length of outer nuclear membranes surveyed was ∼20 μm for each nuclei source.

increase (Table I) indicates that, when rats were treated with PB, P-450(PB) increased without increasing the total cytochrome P-450 content of the nuclear envelope.

This experiment clearly showed that the antigenic sites of cytochrome P-450 molecules do exist on the cytoplasmic side of the outer membrane of the nuclear envelope. It is not clear, however, whether cytochrome P-450 also exists on the nucleoplasmic side of the inner membrane of the nuclear envelope, because ferritin antibody conjugates do not always have free access to this inner nuclear membrane. Hence, the envelopes were isolated by the procedures of Dwyer and Blobel (5) from MC-treated rats and incubated with the ferritin antibody conjugates against P-450(MC). Photo 2A clearly indicates that ferritin particles are attached exclusively to the cytoplasmic side of the outer membrane which is studded with ribosomes.

The nuclear envelopes isolated by the above procedure are occasionally covered by laminal structures, and it is possible that this negative result is simply due to the steric hinderance caused by the presence of these structures. We found that the Golgi fraction prepared according to Hino et al. (12) occasionally contains nuclear envelopes as shown in Photo 2B but that the nucleoplasmic surfaces of these envelopes are not covered by the laminal structures. In Fig. 2B the nucleoplasmic surfaces of the envelopes are again seen not labeled with ferritin. In this figure note the complete absence of ferritin particles on the cisternal surface of the outer membrane (small arrows), which became freely accessible to the antibody conjugates by the detachment of the inner membranes.

In order to examine whether the luminal surface of the inner and outer membranes of the nuclear envelopes is labeled with ferritin, the outer membrane was partially detached from its inner counterpart by mechanical homogenization and the nuclei were then incubated with antibody conjugates. Photo 3 indicates that neither luminal surface is labeled.

From these observations we conclude that cytochrome P-450 in the hepatocyte nuclear envelopes exists exclusively on the cytoplasmic surface of the outer membrane. This means that it does not exist in the inner membrane and that the cytochrome P-450 molecules are either a cytoplasmic side monotopic membrane protein or a transmembrane protein having no antigenic determinant on the luminal surface of the outer membranes.

Nuclear Pores as a Diffusion Barrier of Cytochrome P-450 and Biochemical Heterogeneity of the Outer and Inner Membranes of the Nuclear Envelopes

The observations mentioned above suggest the importance of the nuclear pore as a diffusion barrier of cytochrome P-450. To determine the exact site of this diffusion barrier we examined the nuclear pore complexes in more detail. Photos 4 and 5 show a cross sectional and a tangential view of the nuclear envelope, respectively. In the former, ferritin particles are present as far as the outer annuli of the nuclear pore complexes (arrows) which are decorated with tangles of fine filaments extending to the chromatin-free intranuclear channels.

The spatial relationships are more clearly shown in the tangential section along the surface of a nuclear envelope (Photo 5). The central part of Photo 5 (star) shows chromatin blocks penetrated by intranuclear channels (arrows), while the peripheral part shows cytoplasm containing rough ER. At the intermediate region there are a number of nuclear pores sectioned at various levels. It is evident that ferritin particles are present on the cytoplasmic surface of the outer nuclear membrane as far as the outer annuli, and in places several of these are aligned along the outer rim of the annuli (arrows). We conclude, therefore, that the nuclear pore complex could be a diffusion barrier for cytochrome P-450 molecules between the outer and inner membranes of the nuclear envelopes.

It has been generally accepted that the enzyme profile of the nuclear envelope is similar to that of ER but usually the specific enzyme activities of the former are only one-third or one-half those of ER (*10, 13, 26, 31*). It is therefore very probable that the microsomal-type enzymes in nuclei are associated mostly with the outer nuclear membrane and that the properties of the inner nuclear membrane are quite different. This conclusion is supported by the exclusive localization of cholesterol-filipin complexes in the outer nuclear membrane shown by Kim and Okada (*17*).

Relationship of the Outer Membranes of the Nuclear Envelopes with the ER Membranes

As described above, the biochemical properties of the outer membranes of the nuclear envelopes have been suggested to be very similar to those of the ER membranes. This is supported by a number of electron microscopic observations which have shown the continuity of outer nuclear membranes and rough ER membranes (*1, 7, 8, 29, 30*). Most ultrastructural investigations of the ER-nuclear envelope relationships reported so far have been empirical and no systematic survey has been reported.

Recently we succeeded in preparing a number of prefixed nuclei from rat liver by perfusion with dilute glutaraldehyde (*22*). These nuclei frequently were associated with the rough ER. Systematic survey of a number of such nuclei showed clearly that indeed there is a direct connection between the two membranes (Photo 4). This figure also shows that the smooth, or ribosome-free, parts of the two membranes are extensively stained with ferritin.

Existence of Cytochrome P-450 within the Nuclei

So far, we have shown that cytochrome P-450 does exist in the nuclear envelopes. The important question is whether or not cytochrome P-450 exists within nuclei. Despite several trials, we were unable to obtain any positive evidence showing its existence within the nuclear matrix. This negative result is consistent with the finding of Rogan *et al.* (*24*) that washing of nuclei with a detergent (Triton N-10) removed the nuclear envelopes and, simultaneously, all the nuclear cytochrome P-450.

In the course of this study, however, we occasionally found that internalization of microsomal vesicles sometimes studded with ribosomes occurred when nuclei were incubated with the antibody or control conjugates (Photo 6). Our interpretation of this was that these inclusion bodies are artificially produced by the internalization of the nuclear envelopes or ER membranes (*22*), because they are usually studded with both ribosomes and ferritin particles. This interpretation is presumably correct in most cases, and we assume that most of the previous papers which report the nuclear localization of cytochrome P-450 could be interpreted in this line. However, it is still possible that the internalization of such vesicles occurs *in vivo*. This problem will be discussed in detail in the next section.

Localization of Cytochrome P-450 in Nuclei and Its Possible Significance in Chemical Carcinogenesis

Our quantitative ferritin immunoelectron microscopic study demonstrated the exclusive localization of cytochrome P-450 on the cytoplasmic surface of the outer nuclear membranes. In agreement with Kasper *et al.* (*6*, *14*), it was preferentially induced by treatment with MC, which is mainly responsible for chemical mutagenesis and carcinogenesis (*9*). The cytochrome P-450 in the nuclear envelopes is definitely closer to the nuclear DNA than in the ER, and the proximity of the site of generation of the relatively instable mutagenic metabolites may be significant in determining the extent and nature of DNA alteration. When the nucleus is markedly invaginated, as schematically shown in Fig. 1, the active carcinogens produced by cytochrome P-450 in the nuclear envelopes may be concentrated within the invaginated subcompartments and efficiently incorporated into the nuclear interior. If the half lives of the active ultimate carcinogens are extremely short, however, almost all the active metabolites may be inactivated in the course of intracellular transport from the cytoplasmic surface of the outer nuclear membrane to the nuclear interior. In such a case, the existence of cytochrome P-450 within the nuclei may be extremely significant for chemical carcinogenesis.

We have demonstrated nuclear inclusion bodies containing cytochrome P-450 within the nuclei (Photo 6). As discussed above most of these inclusions may be artifically produced *in vitro*. It has been reported, however, that similar nuclear inclusion bodies frequently appear *in vivo*, especially in the nuclei of tumor cells (*2*), and it is possible that such inclusion bodies also appear in normal cells *in vivo*. In such a

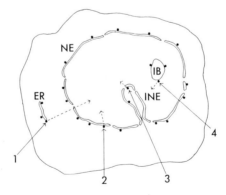

FIG. 1.   Possible routes of transport of precarcinogens and ultimate carcinogens into the nuclear interior. Site of formation of ultimate carcinogens: 1, ER membranes; 2, outer membranes of nuclear envelope (NE); 3, outer membrane of invaginated nuclear envelopes (INE); 4, nuclear inclusion bodies (IB). The small dots indicate cytochrome P-450 molecules, while arrows with continuous and broken lines indicate possible route of transport of precarcinogens and ultimate carcinogens, respectively.

case, the active carcinogens may be produced within the nuclei, which binds directly with DNA, thus inducing malignant transformation. It has been shown that intraperitoneally injected benzo[a]pyrene 7,8-dihydro diol-9,10-epoxide, an active form of benzo[a]pyrene, in newborn Swiss-Webster mice is at least 150 times more effective than benzo[a]pyrene in causing pulmonary and lymphatic tumors (4), and it may be argued that the site of formation of unstable carcinogens is not very important. We must take into consideration, however, that in such *in vitro* experiments far larger amounts of chemical carcinogens are used than we are exposed to in the natural environment. Therefore, morphological changes such as deep invagination of nuclear envelopes and formation of inclusion bodies by internalization of nuclear envelopes or ER membranes containing cytochrome P-450 could play a critical role in the process of chemical carcinogenesis in our natural environment. Figure 1 shows possible routes of transfer of chemical precarcinogens and ultimate procarcinogens into the nuclear interior.

Acknowledgment

This work was partially supported by a Grant-in-Aid for Cancer Research from the Ministry of Education Science and Culture, Japan.

REFERENCES

1. Behnke, O. and H. Moe. An electron microscope study of mature and differentiating Paneth cells in the rat, especially of their endoplasmic reticulum and lysosomes. *J. Cell Biol.*, **22**, 633–652 (1964).

2. Bernhard, W. and Granboulan, N. The fine structure of the cancer cell nucleus. *Exp. Cell Res.* (Suppl. 9), 19–53 (1963).

3. Bresnick, E., Vaught, J. B., Chuang, A.H.L., Stoming, T. A., Bockman, D., and Mukhtar, H. Nuclear aryl hydrocarbon hydroxylase and introduction of polycyclic hydrocarbons with nuclear components. *Arch. Biochem. Biophys.*, **181**, 257–269 (1977).

4. Buening, M. K., Wislocki, P. G., Levin, W., Yagi, H., Thakker, D. R., Akagi, H., Koreeda, M., Jerina, D. M., and Conney, A. H. Tumorigenicity of the optical enantiomers of the diastereomeric benzo(a)pyrene 7,8-diol-9,10-epoxides in newborn mice: Exceptional activity of (+)-7β,8α-dihydroxy-9α,10α-epoxy-7,8,9,10-tetrahydrobenzo(a)pyrene. *Proc. Natl. Acad. Sci. U. S.*, **75**, 5358–5361 (1978).

5. Dwyer, N. and Blobel, G. A modified procedure for isolation of a pore complex lamina fraction from rat liver nuclei. *J. Cell Biol.*, **70**, 581–591 (1976).

6. Fahl, W. E., Jefcoate, C. R., and Kasper, C. B. Characteristics of benzo(a)pyrene metabolism and cytochrome P-450 heterogeneity in rat liver nuclear envelope and comparison to microsomal membrane. *J. Biol. Chem.*, **253**, 3106–3113 (1978).

7. Franke, W. W. and Scheer, U. Structures and functions of the nuclear envelope. *In* "The Cell Nucleus," ed. H. Busch, Vol. 1, pp. 219–347 (1974). Academic Press, New York.

8. Franke, W. W., Scheer, U., Krohne, G., and Jarasch, E.-D. The nuclear envelope and the architecture of the nuclear periphery. *J. Cell Biol.*, **91**, 39S–50S (1981).

9. Hara, E., Kawajiri, K., and Tagashira, Y. Immunochemical study on the contributions of two molecular species of microsomal cytochrome P-450 to the metabolism of benzo(a)pyrene by rat liver microsomes. *Cancer Res.*, **43**, 3604–3608 (1983).

10. Harris, J. R. The biochemistry and ultrastructure of the nuclear envelope. *Biochim. Biophys. Acta*, **515**, 55–104 (1978).

11. Heidelberger, C. Chemical carcinogenesis. *Annu. Rev. Biochem.*, **44**, 79–121 (1975).

12. Hino, Y., Asano, A., and Sato, R. Biochemical studies on rat liver Golgi apparatus. I. Isolation and preliminary characterization. *J. Biochem.*, **83**, 909–923 (1978).

13. Kashing, D. M. and Kasper, C. B. Isolation, morphology, and composition of the nuclear membrane from rat liver. *J. Biol. Chem.*, **244**, 3786–3792 (1969).

14. Kasper, C. B. Biochemical distinctions between the nuclear and microsomal membranes from rat hepatocytes. *J. Biol. Chem.*, **246**, 577–581 (1971).

15. Kawajiri, K., Yonekawa, H., Hara, E., and Tagashira, Y. Activation of 2-acetylaminofluorene in the nuclei of rat liver. *Cancer Res.*, **39**, 1089–1093 (1979).

16. Khandwala, A. S. and Kasper, C. B. Preferential induction of aryl hydroxylase activity in rat liver nuclear envelope by 3-methylcholanthrene. *Biochem. Biophys. Res. Commun.*, **54**, 1241–1246 (1973).

17. Kim, J. and Okada, Y. Asymmetric distribution and temperature-dependent clustering of filipin-sterol complexes in the nuclear membrane of Ehrlich ascites tumor cells. *Eur. J. Cell Biol.*, **29**, 244–252 (1983).

18. Masuda-Mikawa, R., Fujii-Kuriyama, Y., and Tashiro, Y. Purification and partial characterization of hepatic microsomal cytochrome P-450s from phenobarbital- and 3-methylcholanthrene-treated rats. *J. Biochem.*, **86**, 1383–1394 (1979).

19. Matsuura, S., Fujii-Kuriyama, Y., and Tashiro, Y. Immunoelectron microscopic localization of cytochrome P-450 on microsomes and other membrane structures of rat hepatocytes. *J. Cell Biol.*, **78**, 503–519 (1978).

20. Matsuura, S., Fujii-Kuriyama, Y., and Tashiro, Y. Quantitative immunoelectron microscopic analyses of the distribution of cytochrome P-450 molecules on rat liver microsomes. *J. Cell Sci.*, **36**, 413–435 (1979).

21. Matsuura, S., Masuda, R., Omori, K., Negishi, M., and Tashiro, Y. Distribution and induction of cytochrome P-450 in rat liver nuclear envelope. *J. Cell Biol.*, **91**, 212–220 (1981).

22. Matsuura, S., Masuda, R., Sakai, O., and Tashiro, Y. Immunoelectron microscopy of the outer membrane of rat hepatocyte nuclear envelopes in relation to the rough endoplasmic reticulum. *Cell Struct. Funct.*, **8**, 1–19 (1983).

23. Pezzuto, J. M., Lea, M. A., and Yang, C. S. Binding of metabolically activated benzo-(a)pyrene to nuclear macromolecules. *Cancer Res.*, **36**, 3647–3653 (1976).

24. Rogan, E. G., Mailander, P., and Cavalier, E. Metabolic activation of aromatic hydrocarbons in purified rat liver nuclei: Induction of enzyme activities and binding of DNA with and without monooxygenase-catalyzed formation of active oxygen. *Proc. Natl. Acad. Sci. U. S.*, **73**, 457–461 (1976).

25. Rogan, E. G. and Cavalieri, E. 3-methylcholanthrene-inducible binding of aromatic hydrocarbons to DNA in purified rat liver nuclei. *Biochem. Biophys. Res. Commun.*, **58**, 1119–1126 (1974).

26. Sagara, Y., Harano, T., and Omura, T. Characterization of electron transport enzymes in the envelope of rat liver. *J. Biochem.*, **83**, 807–812 (1978).

27. Thomas, P. E., Korzeniowski, D., Bresnick, E., Bornstein, W. A., Kasper, C. B., Fahl, E., Jefcoate, C. R., and Levin, W. Hepatic cytochrome P-448 and epoxide hydrase: Enzymes of nuclear origin are immunochemically identical with those of microsomal origin. *Arch. Biochem. Biophys.*, **192**, 22–26 (1979).

28. Vaught, J. and Bresnick, E. Binding of polycyclic hydrocarbons to nuclear components *in vitro*. *Biochem. Biophys. Res. Commun.*, **69**, 587–591 (1976).

29. Watson, M. L. The nuclear envelope. Its structure and relation to cytoplasmic membranes. *J. Biophys. Biochem. Cytol.*, **1**, 257–270 (1955).

30. Whaley, W. G., Mollenhauer, H. H., and Leech, J. H. Some observations on the nuclear envelope. *J. Biophys. Biochem. Cytol.*, **8**, 233–245 (1960).

31. Zbarsky, I. B. An enzyme profile of the nuclear envelope. *Int. Rev. Cytol.*, **54**, 295–360 (1978).

EXPLANATION OF PHOTOS

PHOTO 1. Rat liver nuclei incubated with anti- P-450(MC) antibody conjugates. Nuclei were prepared from control (A), PB- (B), and MC- (C) treated rat livers, respectively. ×67,500.

PHOTO 2. Rat hepatocyte nuclear envelopes prepared from MC-treated rats by the procedures of (A) Dwyer and Blobel (5), or (B) Hino *et al.* (12) and incubated with anti-P-450(MC). Long arrows, chromatin; short thick arrows, nuclear pores; small arrows, a part of nuclear envelope from which inner nuclear membranes were lost; arrowheads, ribosomes; stars, microsomal vesicles. A, ×80,000; B, ×90,000.

PHOTO 3. Rat liver nuclei prepared from MC-treated rats were homogenized in a tight Teflon glass homogenizer and incubated with anti- P-450(MC) antibody conjugates. O, outer nuclear membrane; I, inner nuclear membrane. Arrowheads indicate nuclear pore complexes and small patches of the outer nuclear membrane still associated with the inner nuclear membranes. ×65,000.

PHOTO 4. Ferritin immunoelectron microscopy of a rough ER in continuity with the outer nuclear membrane. Prefixed nuclei were prepared from MC-treated rats and then incubated with ferritin anti-P-450(MC) antibody conjugates. Arrows: intranuclear chromatin-free channels which are connected to the nuclear pore complexes; arrow-heads: marked labeling with ferritin particles along the outer annuli of the nuclear pore complexes. ×66,000.

PHOTO 5. Tangential view of a nucleus incubated with ferritin anti-P-450(MC). (Explanation in text.) ×75,000.

PHOTO 6. Small vesicles (stars) within the nuclear interior which probably were derived from ER membranes or from the outer nuclear membranes. Unfixed nuclei were prepared from PB-treated rat livers and incubated with ferritin antibody conjugates against P-450(PB). In this figure, a part of the outer nuclear membrane is detached from its inner counterpart (arrow). Neither the outer nor the inner nuclear membrane luminal surface was stained with ferritin. ×88,000.

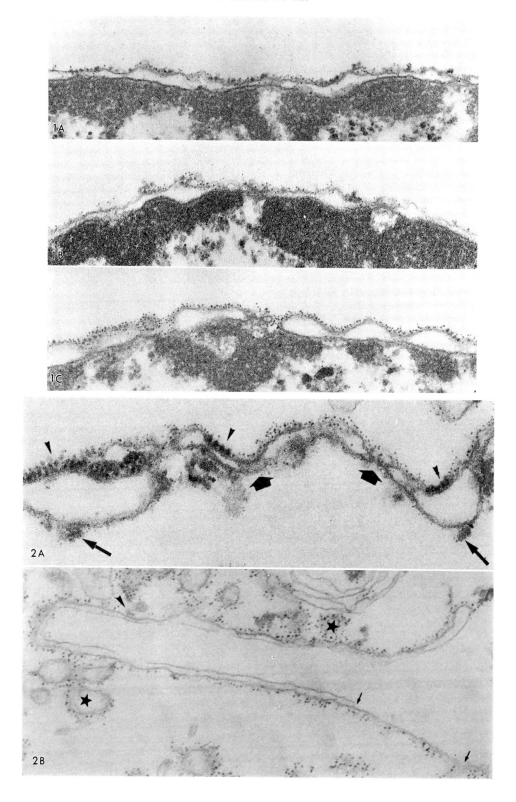

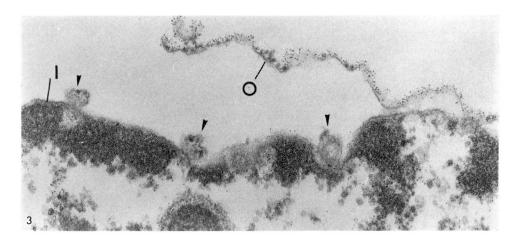

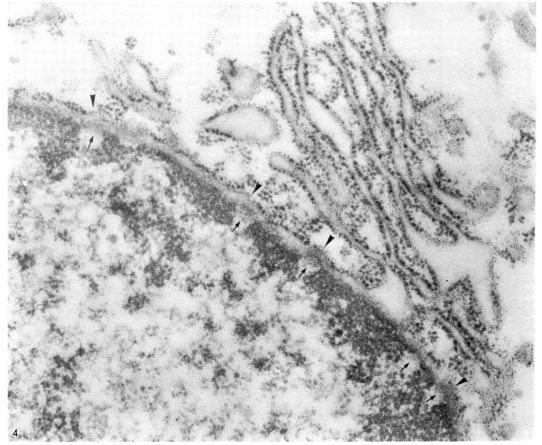

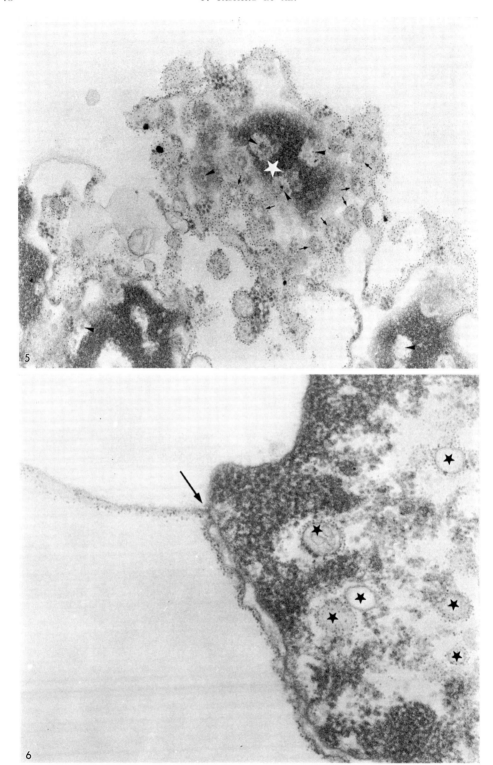

MICROSOMAL CYTOCHROME P-450 IN HIGHER PLANTS

Ken HIGASHI

*Department of Biochemistry, School of Medicine, University of Occupational and Environmental Health**

Studies involving the metabolism of xenobiotics in plants are important with regard to the human food chain and public health. The occurrence of cytochrome P-450 in the microsomes of various higher plants has been reported by many investigators. The mechanism of cytochrome P-450-catalyzed reactions in plants, however, has not been characterized as thoroughly as the hepatic microsomal enzymes. The optical and magnetic characteristics of plant cytochrome P-450 preparations closely resemble those of hepatic microsomes. NADPH is a major source of electrons for reduction of cytochrome P-450 in plants as in liver microsomes. In general, the plant cytochrome P-450 systems may have a much narrower specificity for substrates than is found in the cytochrome P-450 species from liver. It is unknown whether a system equivalent to the drug-induced hepatic mono-oxygenase having a broad specificity is present in higher plants.

Much information now exists in regard to the metabolic fate of organic pesticides and herbicides in plants, but many of the metabolic data available have their origin in mode-of-action studies (*8*). A new topic has arisen involving the metabolism of xenobiotics in plants or field detoxication mechanism. Possible activations of innocuous chemicals into mutagens by the plant enzymatic system should be considered for both environmental conservation and the human food chain.

Presumably, many of the environmental chemicals are biotransformed by plants in a manner similar to those of the mammalian microsomal activation system, which is employed in short-term microbial assay. There are, however, only a few instances in the literature where mutagenicity data from higher plant assays have been compared with data from other non-mammalian and mammalian assays (*10*). Although a number of agents are activated by both plants and animals into mutagens, some appear to be activated only by plants (*40*).

With regard to the human food chain and public health, the need has arisen for (a) a systematic survey of various plant species to determine the comparative biochemistry of activation and detoxication mechanisms and (b) active *in vitro* systems capable of at least qualitatively reproducing the reactions which occur in living plants, particularly microsomal cytochrome P-450 from higher plants. This review is concerned only with data of microsomal cytochrome P-450 from higher plants; such data is sparse because only a comparatively few groups are investigating this subject,

---

* Iseigaoka 1-1, Yahata Nishi-ku, Kitakyushu, Fukuoka 870, Japan (東　監).

though mammalian cytochrome P-450 is better researched. *In vivo* metabolism of environmental chemicals by plants is not dealt with here.

Occurrence of Cytochrome P-450 in Plants

In 1969, Frear *et al.* (*13*) confirmed the presence of mixed function oxidase in the extract from etiolated cotton seedling hypocotyls. The enzyme catalyzed N-demethylation of substituted 3-(phenyl)-1-methylurea and required the presence of oxygen molecules, NADPH, cytochrome b_5 and NADPH-cytochrome *c* reductase. The enzyme system was inhibited by thiol reagents, chelating reagents, electron acceptors, and carbon monoxide, however, direct evidence for the presence of a P-450-type cytochrome has not been found. The mixed function oxidase in tissue homogenates of *Echinocystis macrocarpa* Greene endosperm, on the other hand, has been observed by Murphy and West (*37*) and the conversion of (−)-kaur-16-en-19-aldehyde to (−)-kaur-16-en-19-oic acid was inhibited by carbon monoxide. The photochemical action spectrum for this reaction showed a maximum reversal at 450 nm. Later, Markham *et al.* (*33*) reported the presence of cytochrome P-450-like pigments in microsomes from *Phaseolus vulgaris* (bean) cotyledons, *Pisum sativum* (pea) seedlings, and *Zea mais* (maize) cotyledons.

Subsequently, the optical and magnetic properties of the cytochrome P-450 in microsomes from a variety of higher plants have been studied (*45, 46*). On the basis of binding studies with ethylisocyanide, degradation of cytochrome P-450 to P-420, redox potential, and relative rates of reduction by NADPH and NADH, it was suggested that the cytochrome P-450 system in higher plants is analogous to that in mammalian microsomes. The technique of electron paramagnetic resonance spectrophotometry has been applied to study the microsomal electron transport components of tulip (*Tulipa gesneriana* L.) bulbs (*46*). At 77K in the oxidized state, signals at $g=2.40$, 2.25, and 1.93, characteristic of cytochrome P-450 in the low-spin state, and also at $g=4.27$, attributable to ferric iron in a rhombic environment, were observed. The signals at $g=2.40$, 2.25, and 1.93 disappeared upon reduction with sodium dithionite. At 10°K in the oxidized state, signals at $g=8.3$ and 3.3 appeared, and these were attributed to high-spin cytochrome P-450.

Fractionation of plant cell extracts by differential centrifugation does not achieve a clean separation of organelle fractions; microsomal fraction also contains fragmented dictyosomes, tonoplasts, and plasma membranes. A better way to isolate the endoplasmic reticulum from plant cells is by sucrose density gradient centrifugation. When the tissue is homogenized in a medium containing 1 mM EDTA, the endoplasmic reticulum bands at a density of 1.11–1.12 g/cm³ (*29*). Homogenates from germinating castor bean (*Recinus communis var.* Hale) endosperm were fractionated for mixed function oxidase (*10*). Activity of cinnamate 4-hydroxylase and *p*-chloro-N-methylaniline N-demethylase was highest in the endoplasmic reticulum fraction with equilibrium density 1.12 g/cm³. Activity of both enzymes is dependent on NADPH and molecular oxygen and both are inhibited by carbon monoxide.

On the other hand, the intracellular location of a cytochrome P-450-dependent monoterpene hydroxylase from *Catharanthus roseus* G. Don (*Vinca roseus*) has been investigated by Madyastha *et al.* (*32*). By differential and sucrose density gradient

TABLE I. Cytochrome P-450 Content in the Microsomes of Various Plant Tissues

Source	Cytochrome P-450 (nmol/mg protein)
Cauliflower bud	
Uninduced	0.051 (0.04–0.07) [b]
Induced [a]	0.085 (0.06–0.10)
Potato	
Uninduced	(—) [c]
Induced	0.055 (0.056, 0.054)
Jerusalem artichoke	
Uninduced	0.015 (0.012–0.017)
Induced	0.141 (0.126–0.157)
Symplocarpus spadix	0.058
Avocado mesocarp	0.316 (0.221–0.458)
Tulip bulb	0.320 (0.204–0.488)

[a] Incubated for 14–18 hr after slicing.
[b] Range of values determined.
[c] Too low to be determined.

centrifugation, utilizing marker enzymes and electron microscopy, the monooxygenase was demonstrated to be associated with vesicles having a density of 1.09 to 1.10 g/cm^3; these vesicles could be distinguished from endoplasmic reticulum. The results suggest that at least one of the first steps in the biosynthesis of indole alkaloids might be compartmentalized (11).

In our laboratory, microsomal fractions were prepared from appropriate tissues of various plants and their cytochrome P-450 contents were determined (Table I). These values were somewhat varied in different experiments due to the differences of time after harvesting or conditions of storage (24). The individual values of cytochrome P-450 content in a single tissue, however, did not differ significantly beyond a certain point and individual plant tissues had distinct ranges. The profiles of carbon monoxide difference spectra of plant microsomes from uninduced materials frequently showed greater amounts of P-420 than P-450, though only the content of P-450 is calculated in Table I. After incubation of potato and Jerusalem artichoke tuber discs and sliced fragments of cauliflower buds, an increase of cytochrome P-450 was observed, as described later. Compared with those of induced sources of Jerusalem artichoke, potato and cauliflower, microsomes of both tulip bulbs and avocado mesocarps contained a large quantity of cytochrome P-450 but little P-420, even without treatment.

Cytochrome P-450 Dependent Metabolism

1. Cinnamate 4-monooxygenase

In higher plants, phenylalanine is metabolized to *trans*-cinnamic acid by phenylalanine ammonia-lyase (EC 4.3.1.5) and then this product is converted to 4-hydroxycinnamic acid by *trans*-cinnamate 4-monooxygenase (EC 1.13.14.11). Since 4-hydroxycinnamic acid is situated at a branch point in the biosynthesis of many phenolic compounds, the majority of these compounds must possess a hydroxyl group in a position corresponding to carbon atom 4 of the cinnamic acid-derived moiety (60). Russell and Conn in 1967 have showed the presence of the enzyme catalyzing the step of *trans*-

cinnamic acid to 4-hydroxycinnamic acid (*p*-coumaric acid) in the extract of apical buds of pea seedlings (*48*). They found NADPH and tetrahydrofolic acid were required for this hydroxylation. However, a further report on the pea seedling enzyme (*49*) revealed that the presence of 2-mercaptoethanol in the tetrahydrofolic acid solution enhanced this reaction. The studies by Russell (*49*) have shown that this enzyme is located in the microsomal fraction and is required for NADPH and molecular oxygen. Furthermore, conversion of *trans*-cinnamate to 4-hydroxycinnamate was inhibited by carbon monoxide and reversed by light. The action spectra for light reversal peaked at 450 nm, confirming the participation of a P-450 type of cytochrome in this reaction.

Further investigations of 4-hydroxylation of *trans*-cinnamate have been carried out with sorghum seedlings (*41*), aged swede root discs (*21*), castor bean endosperm (*59*), washed potato slices (*47*), Jerusalem artichoke tubers (*4*), pea seedlings (*5*), and gherkin tissues (*7*). These studies confirmed the requirements of NADPH and molecular oxygen. The induction of *trans*-cinnamate 4-hydroxylase activity during aging was shown to be roughly proportional to the increase of cytochrome P-450 content in the microsomes of wounded tissues of Jerusalem artichoke (*4*).

2. Kaurene oxidation

Kaurene is a precursor of plant growth-regulating gibberellins. Two of the initial reactions in the oxidative conversion of (−)-kaurene-16-ene to gibberellin have been studied in tissue homogenates of *E. macrocarpus* Greene (wild cucumber) endosperm (*37*). The conversions of both (−)-kaur-16-ene to (−)-kaur-16-en-19-ol and (−)-kaur-16-en-19-aldehyde to (−)-kaur-16-en-19-oic acid require oxygen and NADPH and are inhibited by carbon monoxide. The photochemical action spectrum for these reactions showed a maximal reversal at 450 nm, as described in the preceding section. The conversion of kaurenol to kaurenal was inhibited by NADP⁺, *p*-chloromercuribenzoate and β-diethyl aminoethyldiphenylvalerate dihydrochloride (SKF-525A). These properties suggest kaurene oxidation is catalyzed by mixed function oxidases (*11*).

Furthermore, Hasson and West (*17*) attempted to solubilize cytochrome P-450 and other electron transport components from microsomes prepared from endosperm tissues of immature *Marah macrocarpus* (*E. macrocarpus*) seeds. They confirmed the presence of cytochrome b_5, NADH-cytochrome *c* reductase and NADPH-cytochrome *c* reductase by partial separation of these components with DEAE-cellulose column chromatography. Their data suggested the possible component participation in the mixed function oxidation of kaurene. It seems the cytochrome P-450-dependent mixed function oxidations in higher plant systems have many features in common with hepatic microsomal cytochrome P-450-dependent oxidase.

3. Abscisic acid metabolism

A cell-free enzyme system capable of metabolizing abscisic acid has been obtained by Gillard and Walton (*14*), from Eastern wild cucumber (*Echinocystis lobata* Michx.) liquid endosperm. The products were determined to be phaseic acid and dihydrophaseic acid. The dihydrophaseic acid pathway has a role in regulating the hormonal activity of abscisic acid, such as growth inhibition and abscission promotion. This particulate abscisic acid hydroxylating enzyme showed a requirement for oxygen and NADPH and inhibition by carbon monoxide. Unlike many of the rat liver microsomal monooxygenases, the abscisic acid hydroxylating enzyme has a high substrate specificity for (+)-abscisic acid. The (−)-abscisic acid is only 1/10 as effective a substrate as the naturally occurring (+)-abscisic acid. In the case of t,t-(±)-abscisic acid, (±)-abscisic acid methyl ester, and the 1′,4′-diols of (±)-abscisic acid, no reaction products were determined (14).

4. Monoterpene hydroxylase

Meehan and Coscia (35) reported on a microsomal preparation from V. rosea seedlings capable of hydroxylating both geraniol and nerol specifically at the C-10 methyl group. Light reversible inhibition by carbon monoxide as well as differential sensitivity to other inhibitors established the hydroxylase as a cytochrome P-450 type. Geraniol hydroxylation was enhanced by dithiothreitol and inhibited by phospholipases, thiol reagents, metyrapone, and cytochrome c. The membrane bound hydroxylase was solubilized by treatment with sodium cholate and resolved by DEAE-cellulose chromatography (31). A good separation of the fractions rich in P-450 heme protein from the NADPH-cytochrome c reductase was achieved with this chromatography. Optimal activity was observed with a combination of reductase, heme protein, and lipid extract. However, the reconstituted system yielded only 10–15% of the hydroxylase activity present in the solubilized membrane fraction probably due to the highly labile nature of the cytochrome P-450. But this partial success is only one instance of the reconstituted monooxygenase system from higher plant sources. The results at least indicate that the plant enzyme is dependent on cytochrome P-450, NADPH-cytochrome c reductase and lipid for activity, as is true in hepatic microsomal enzymes.

5. Hydroxylation of fatty acids

ω-Hydroxylation of fatty acids, which is a key reaction in the biosynthesis of cutin and suberin, was demonstrated for the first time by Soliday and Kolattukudy (25, 54, 55) in a microsomal fraction from germinating embryonic shoots of Vicia faba. This enzymic hydroxylation required molecular oxygen and NADPH, but substitution of NADH resulted in nearly half of the reaction rate obtained with NADPH. As expected of a hydroxylase involving cytochrome P-450, the ω-hydroxylation was inhibited by carbon monoxide and the enzyme system showed unusually high sensitivity to this inhibition; 10% CO caused some inhibition and 30% CO completely inhibited the reaction.

Exogenous labeled palmitic acid was first hydroxylated at the ω-position and subsequently at C-10 before being incorporated into cutin (55). This mid-chain hydroxylation also required molecular oxygen and NADPH and was inhibited by NaN_2, metal ion chelators such as O-phenanthroline and 8-hydroxyquinoline, and thiol-directed reagents such as N-ethylmaleimide and p-chloromercuribenzoate. Photoreversible inhibition of the mid-chain hydroxylation by carbon monoxide suggested the involvement of a cytochrome P-450 type protein. Drastic differences in the sensitivity to carbon monoxide and photoreversibility of this inhibition suggest that ω-hydroxylation and mid-chain hydroxylation are catalyzed by two different enzymes.

A lauric acid monooxygenase which catalyzes the formation of hydroxylaurate from lauric acid has been demonstrated by Salaün et al. (51) in aging tissues of Jerusalem artichoke (Helianthus tuberosus L.) tuber. NADPH-cytochrome c reductase is involved in electron transfer as evidenced by the inhibitory effects of NADP$^+$ and oxidized cytochrome c on laurate monooxygenase.

6. Exogenous compounds

Etiolated cotton hypocotyl microsomal preparations were able to readily N-de-methylate several substituted 3-(phenyl)-1-methylurea compounds, such as 3-(3,4-dichlorophenyl)-1,1-dimethylurea, 3-(3-trifluoromethylphenyl)-1,1-dimethylurea, 3-(4-chlorophenyl)-1,1-dimethylurea(Monuron), and 3-(4-chlorophenyl)-1-methylurea, but did not function with N,N-dimethyl-2,2-diphenylacetamide or 2-chloro-4-ethylamino-6-isopropylamino-s-triazine, which have been reported to be dealkylated by *in vivo* plant systems. Under the assay conditions used in these studies, the cotton microsomal N-demethylase system appeared to be specific for substituted 3-(phenyl)-1-methyl-urea substrates (13). Frear *et al.* (13) have also isolated active N-demethylase preparations from plantin, buckwheat, wild buckwheat, and broadbeans.

Inhibition studies with the cotton microsomal N-demethylase system were carried out to examine the mechanism for N-demethylation of substituted 3-(phenyl)-1-methyl-ureas. Studies with a number of substituted N-methylcarbamates showed that a high electron density at the ortho position relative to the carbamate group was necessary for an effective inhibition of N-demethylation. Similar studies with several substituted phenylureas demonstrated that the proton on the aniline nitrogen atom was also neces-sary for effective inhibition of the microsomal N-demethylation system (57).

Activity of *p*-chloro-N-methylaniline N-demethylase in the endoplasmic reticulum fraction of castor bean endosperm is dependent on NADPH and on molecular oxygen; this activity was inhibited by carbon monoxide (59). In the absence of NADPH, cumen hydroperoxide was able to support N-demethylation. Aminopyrine N-demethylation was found to increase in Jerusalem artichoke tuber tissues by inducers that also stimulate *trans*-cinnamate 4-hydroxylase activity. The increase in this N-demethylase activity roughly paralleled that of cytochrome P-450. Although light reversal of CO-inhibition was not carried out in this case (6), the data described in this section strongly suggest that cytochrome P-450 in higher plants is capable of at least the N-demethylation of xenobiotics.

Induction of Cytochrome P-450

Resting plant storage organs such as carrots, red beets, sugar beets or potato tubers can be activated by slicing them into thin discs and incubating these fragments in a moist atmosphere for different periods of time ("aging") (56). Phenylalanine ammonia-lyase in potato-, sweet potato-, swede-, and Jerusalem artichoke discs in-creased after slicing them and showed a maximum level enzyme activity approximately 30 hr later (22, 61). Electron microscopic observations of intact tissues of Jerusalem artichoke showed that rudimentary endoplasmic reticulum and dictyosomes were practically absent in these resting tubers. Rough endoplasmic reticulum increased significantly 24 hr after wounding, accompanied by a considerably increased capacity of protein synthesis when compared with fractions from fresh tissue slices (56).

Cinnamate 4-monooxygenase, a key enzyme in phenylpropanoid biosynthesis, is located on the endoplasmic reticulum and can be induced by slicing in Jerusalem

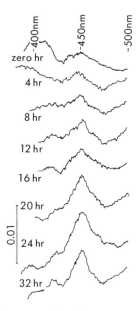

FIG. 1. Changes of carbon monoxide-difference spectrum of microsomes during incubation of Jerusalem artichoke tuber slices. Approximately 8 g of slices was used for each time point. Microsomes were suspended in 0.1 M sodium phosphate buffer, pH 7.4, containing 28% glycerol (*18*).

artichoke tuber tissues (*4*). The induction and subsequent changes of cinnamate 4-monooxygenase activity during aging are accounted for by the variation in NADPH-cytochrome *c* reductase and cytochrome P-450 content (*4*). The content of cytochrome b_5, already present in the dormant tuber, is also markedly enhanced by wounding.

The changes of CO-difference spectra of microsomes during the incubation of Jerusalem artichoke tuber discs (*18*) are shown in Fig. 1. Discs (0.5–1.0 mm thick) were vigorously shaken in flasks in distilled water at 25°C in the dark; after a given period of aging, microsomes were prepared as described previously (*18*). In the quiescent tubers (0 hr in Fig. 1), the peak at 450 nm was not as sharp as those of induced preparations and the amount of absorbance at around 420 nm was significant. The height of the 450 nm peak increased gradually with time and reached a plateau 20–24 hr after the start of incubation. Absorbance around 420 nm decreased and became negative in the later period of incubation. It is unknown yet whether the disappearance of absorbance around 420 nm is due to degradation of the heme protein itself or to the release of the heme moiety from apoprotein. The increase of cytochrome P-450 in endoplasmic reticulum was less significant in older Jerusalem artichoke tubers.

Increase of microsomal cytochrome P-450 after wounding was also detected in cauliflower buds (Table I), but no increase was observed in slices of tulip bulbs (data not shown here). The latter tissues contained relatively high levels of microsomal cytochrome even in the uninduced state (Table I).

The involvement of light in the regulation of the biosynthesis of flavonoids and their precursors, the phenylpropanoids, is well known (*2, 15*). The biosynthetic pathway contained phenylalanine ammonia-lyase and *trans*-cinnamate 4-monooxygenase in its early steps. Benveniste *et al.* (*5*) observed the stimulation by light of *trans*-cinnamate

4-monooxygenase in dark germinating pea seedlings, although its specific activity increased by only 30%; a slight stimulation of cytochrome P-450 concentration was also observed. In the pea seedling apical buds, both blue and red lights are effective in promoting this enzyme activity: The involvement of phytochrome in the regulation of the enzyme was demonstrated by the red-far red photo-reversion observed on *trans*-cinnamate 4-monooxygenase activity.

Furthermore, blue light mediates a transient increase in the extractable activity of phenylalanine ammonia-lyase from both cotyledons and hypocotyls of etiolated gherkin seedlings, but concurrent changes in extractable *trans*-cinnamate 4-monooxygenase activity only occur in cotyledons. Excision, followed by incubation in the dark, also results in stimulation of the lyase activity in both tissues, but the monooxygenase activity is only stimulated in cotyledons, again concurrently with the lyase. These results indicate that the induction of the two enzymes is tissue-specific and regulated independently (7).

Many of the investigations of mammalian microsomal cytochrome P-450 have been carried out after induction by appropriate inducers, such as phenobarbital, methylcholanthrene, and Aroclor. However, little information was available about the inducers of the plant cytochrome P-450 system until recently, except wounding and light as cited above. Reichhart *et al.* (43) have reported recently that in wound-induced Jerusalem artichoke tissues the cytochrome P-450 content is strongly enhanced by manganese, iron, ethanol, phenobarbital, and several herbicides. The outline of their experiments is as follows:

One-millimeter-thick slices were incubated in the dark at 25°C in flasks with distilled water and vigorously shaken to maintain sufficient aeration. Both the activity of *trans*-cinnamate 4-monooxygenase and cytochrome P-450 content simultaneously reached a maximum 24 hr after slicing and declined thereafter (43). The effects of several substances were examined in this system. The highest effect of ethanol was produced by 300 mM concentration; other alcohols were also effective (methanol, isopropanol). Phenobarbital was a weak inducer of cytochrome P-450 at a concentration of 4 mM stimulating an increase in the content of only 45% as compared with the content of control (distilled water alone) samples at 24 hr. Manganese, 25 mM, was a good inducer of cytochrome P-450 content and *trans*-cinnamate 4-monooxygenase. Iron alone did not alter the levels of cytochrome P-450 in water-aged tissues but enhanced significantly the effect of manganese. 3-(4-Chlorophenyl)-1,1-dimethylurea (Monuron) and 2,6-dichlorobenzonitrile (Dichlobenil), enhanced the cytochrome P-450 content by 100% and 40%, respectively. Thirty percent stimulation of *trans*-cinnamate 4-monooxygenase was detected only with Dichlobenil.

The time courses of induction of cytochrome P-450 and other microsomal electron transporting components were studied in more detail by the same authors (44). In tissues exposed to manganese, biphasic induction patterns of *trans*-cinnamate monooxygenase and cytochrome P-450 were observed. In the first 24 hr, the effect of metal superimposed that produced by wounding alone. Both *trans*-cinnamate 4-monooxygenase and cytochrome P-450 continued to increase in the presence of manganese, reached maximum 70–90 hr after the start of incubation and decreased thereafter. NADPH-cytochrome c reductase was not enhanced by manganese but rather time-shifted, the maximum being reached after 48 hr. Cytochrome b_5 was considerably less induced by manganese than cytochrome P-450. On the contrary, when tissues were exposed to 4 mM phenobarbital, cytochrome P-450 reached a maximum 60 hr after slicing and its pattern was not exactly parallel with that of *trans*-cinnamate 4-mono-oxygenase. This could be due to the heterogeneity of new cytochrome P-450 species. The activity of NADPH-cytochrome c reductase was enhanced 50% by phenobarbital, while b_5 was not significantly affected by this drug.

Similar studies have been carried out with 2,4-dichloro-phenoxyacetate (2,4-D) and Jerusalem artichoke tubers (1). Interestingly, the activities of the in-chain hydroxylation of lauric acid, of NADPH-cytochrome c reductase and the titer of cytochrome b_5 were not substantially altered, whereas *trans*-cinnamate 4-monooxygenase, NADH-cytochrome c reductase and cytochrome P-450 content were significantly enhanced. These results indicated that the enhancement of induction was selective at the level of different redox components and hydroxylase enzymes.

Multiplicity of Cytochrome P-450

Recently, we prepared microsomes from cauliflower (*Brassica oleracea*) buds, potato (*Solanum tuberosum*) tubers, avocado (*Persea americana*) mesocarps, tulip (*Tulipa gesneriana*) bulbs, and Jerusalem artichoke (*Helianthus tuberosus*) tubers and their cytochrome P-450 contents and *trans*-cinnamate 4-monooxygenase were determined (24). The contents of cytochrome P-450 in microsomes of these tissues is listed in Table I. Using these microsomes, we determined *trans*-cinnamate 4-monooxygenase activities (Table II) by radioactive assay as described by Potts *et al.* (41). Activity of this enzyme in microsomes of artichoke tubers increased parallel with the cytochrome P-450 content after wounding, as described by others (4, 44). Microsomes from both avocado mesocarps and tulip bulbs have similar levels of cytochrome P-450 contents and similar carbon monoxide difference spectra (P-448 type), but the *trans*-cinnamate 4-monooxygenase activity of avocado microsomes was approximately 20-fold higher than that of tulip bulbs. On the contrary, little *trans*-cinnamate 4-monooxygenase

TABLE II. Activity of *trans*-Cinnamate 4-Monooxygenase in the Microsomes of Various Plant Tissues

Source	*trans*-Cinnamate 4-monooxygenase	
	HCHO nmol/mg protein	HCHO nmol/nmol P-450
Cauliflower bud		
Uninduced	0.003	0.05 (0.03%)[b]
Induced[a]	0.003	0.05 (0.03%)
Potato tuber		
Induced	10.2	185.4 (100%)
Jerusalem artichoke		
Uninduced	0.1	6.6 (3.6%)
Induced	1.1	7.8 (4.2%)
Avocado mesocarp	6.5	20.0 (10.8%)
Tulip bulb	0.3	0.9 (0.5%)

[a] Incubated for 14–18 hr after slicing.
[b] The value for potato is designated as 100%.

activity was detected in microsomes prepared from either uninduced or induced
cauliflower buds. The highest specific activity of the enzyme was observed in potato
microsomes, although the levels of cytochrome P-450 in both cauliflower and potato
microsomes are similar. These results suggest that there exists a *trans*-cinnamate specific
form of cytochrome P-450 in plant microsomes and *trans*-cinnamate 4-monooxygenase
activity in individual tissues which are not always proportional to the total content of
microsomal cytochrome P-450.

There are, however, two possibilities regarding the multiplicity of cytochrome
P-450 in higher plants: First, each individual plant tissue contains a single form of
cytochrome P-450 and each has a different turnover number for cinnamate; secondly,
individual tissues have multiple forms of cytochrome P-450 and the distribution of
each form is different. Accumulated data suggest that the second possibility is more
likely.

Salaün *et al.* (*52*) compared the products of the laurate hydroxylase in the microsomes prepared from Jerusalem artichoke tuber tissues and apical buds of pea seedlings.
Surprisingly, the tuber tissue enzyme hydroxylates in the chain exclusively, while the
pea seedling enzyme is an ω-hydroxylase. The ω-laurate hydroxylase also differed from
in-chain laurate hydroxylase through its lower specific activity and relatively high
reaction rates sustained by NADH when given alone. Induction of the microsomal
cytochrome P-450 system by wounding the tuber tissues was further enhanced when
the aging medium was supplemented with manganese ions. In the presence of manganese, *trans*-cinnamate 4-monooxygenase increased three times over the water control,
but in-chain laurate hydroxylase was stimulated 100 times. The two monooxygenase
enzymes in a single tissue are regulated independently, and therefore catalyzed by
different cytochrome P-450.

Induction of in-chain laurate hydroxylase by wounding is weak and remains stable
at a low level for at least 120 hr, while that of *trans*-cinnamate 4-monooxygenase is
significant when submitted to the same treatment. In tissues exposed to manganese,
however, laurate in-chain hydroxylase was strongly stimulated as described above.
The effect of phenobarbital treatment on laurate in-chain-hydroxylase was greater
than that of manganese, while the reverse situation was observed for *trans*-cinnamate
4-monooxygenase (*53*). This laurate in-chain hydroxylase appeared strictly specific
for the C-12 free fatty acid and produced predominantly C-9 derivative. These two
monooxygenases showed independent induction and regulation patterns, suggesting the
heterogeneity of cytochrome P-450 in higher plants.

The catalytic self-destruction of hepatic microsomal cytochrome P-450 during the
metabolism of certain types of substrates, including olefins (*38*) and 1-aminobenzotria-
zole (*34*), has recently been documented. Incubation of microsomes of Jerusalem
artichoke with 1-aminobenzotriazole results in time-dependent autocatalytic inactivation of *trans*-cinnamate 4-monooxygenase (*34*). Cytochrome b_5 and NADPH-cytochrome c reductase are not affected. Lauric acid hydroxylase is decreased at a much
slower rate than cinnamate 4-hydroxylase. The results suggest that 1-aminobenzotriazole
is a selective suicide substrate for cinnamate 4-monooxygenase in this plant tissue.

Molecular Properties

No purified preparation of plant cytochrome P-450 had been obtained due to the difficulty of isolating organella and enzymes from higher plant tissues because of the rigid cell wall, the presence of phenolic compounds (*28*) and low concentration of microsomal cytochrome P-450 (*45*). However, we have recently succeeded in isolating an almost electrophoretically homogeneous preparation (more than 98%) of cytochrome P-450 from the microsomes of tulip bulbs (*20*). The procedure employed for purification of cytochrome P-450 from tulip bulbs was essentially the same as that for rat liver microsomes (*50*). In other words, the physical property of plant cytochrome P-450 during column chromatography resembled that of rat liver.

The steps and techniques used to purify cytochrome P-450 from tulip bulb-

TABLE III. Purification of Microsomal Cytochrome P-450 from Tulip Bulbs

Purification step	Total protein (mg)	Total P-450 (nmol)	Specific content (nmol/mg prot.)	Yield[a] (%)
Solubilized fraction	1,540	342.5	0.222	100
DEAE-Sephadex A-52 column chromatography	811.5	100.9	0.124	29.5
Polyethylene glycol Ppt.	266.0	60.9	0.229	17.8
DEAE-cellulose (DE-52) column chromatography	26.9	34.6	1.286	10.1
Hydroxyapatite column chromatography	3.74	25.0	6.684	7.3

[a] Yield represents the percent of cytochrome P-450 recovered at each step from the total content of cytochrome P-450 present in solubilized fractions but not in microsomes.

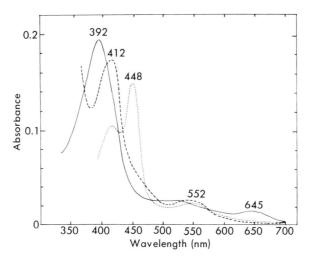

FIG. 2. Absorption spectra of purified cytochrome P-450 preparation from microsomes of tulip bulbs (unpublished data). The solvent was 10 mM potassium phosphate buffer, pH 7.25, containing 0.5% sodium cholate, 0.2% Emulgen 911, 1 mM EDTA, 0.1 mM dithiothreitol, and 20% glycerol. —— oxidized form; ---- reduced with dithionite; ······ carbon monoxide complex.

TABLE IV. Amino Acid Composition of Purified Cytochrome P-450 from
Tulip Bulbs and Rat Livers (20)

	Tulip bulbs		Rat livers[a]	
	No. of residues	%	No. of residues	%
Asx	48	10.0	41	8.8
Thr	27	5.6	26	5.6
Ser	37	7.7	31	6.6
Glx	42	8.8	46	9.9
Pro	36	7.5	27	5.8
Gly	42	8.8	36	7.7
Ala	36	7.5	25	5.4
Cys/2	5	1.0	6	1.3
Val	34	7.0	27	5.8
Met	7	1.5	11	2.4
Ile	19	4.0	26	5.6
Leu	45	9.4	53	11.3
Tyr	16	3.3	14	3.0
Phe	29	6.0	31	6.6
Lys	39	8.1	29	6.2
His	7	1.5	13	2.8
Arg	20	4.2	23	4.9
Trp	ND	—	2	0.4
Total	480		467	
Asx, Glx		18.8		18.7
Arg, Lys, His		13.8		13.9
Gly, Ala, Val, Leu, Ile		36.7		35.8
Phe, Tyr, (Trp)		9.3		10.0

[a] Means of 12 determinations reported.
ND, not determined.

microsomes are summarized in Table III. This procedure results in 7% recovery of the purified cytochrome P-450 present in the solubilized microsomes. The purity of the cytochrome P-450 preparation was investigated by SDS-polyacrylamide gel electrophoresis (27). The purified cytochrome P-450 migrated as a single band (20) essentially free of other contaminants; its molecular weight was calculated as 52,500. The absolute spectra of oxidized form, reduced form by dithionite, and the CO-complex of the reduced form (Fig. 2) are similar to those reported with rat livers (50). The amino acid composition of purified cytochrome P-450 indicates that the protein contains 41% hydrophobic residues and, in general, resembles the average values of 12 different data of rat liver-cytochrome P-450 (Table IV). Characterization of purified cytochrome P-450 from tulip bulbs showed a close relationship to the same hemeprotein groups of animal tissues.

Next, we prepared anti-P-450 serum after injections into rabbits of the mixture of purified cytochrome P-450 and Freund's complete adjuvant. The antibodies against cytochrome P-450 of tulip bulbs were purified by cytochrome P-450-Sepharose 4B column. Microsomes from various plants listed in Table I were analyzed after solubilization in the same buffer used in solubilizing those of tulip bulbs during purification. Antibodies against purified cytochrome P-450 from tulip bulbs formed a single precipitin line with either crude extract of the microsomes from tulip bulbs or purified preparation of the antigen of substance (20). However, no precipitin line was detected with solubilized preparations of microsmes from Jerusalem artichoke tubers, potato tubers, avocado mesocarps or cauliflower buds. Microsomes from induced Jerusalem artichoke failed to show an immunoprecipitin line (data not shown).

Accordingly, we attempted to examine the microsomes from other related plant species. None of the microsomes from bulbs of lily (*Lilium lancifolium*), allium (*Allium shoenoprasum*), narcissus (*Narcissus tazetta*) or gladiolus (*Gladiolus gandavensis*) shared any antigenicity with purified cytochrome P-450 from tulip bulbs, although there existed comparable amounts of cytochrome P-450 in these microsomes (data not shown). We have not yet examined the catalytic activities of purified cytochrome P-450 for different substrates with reconstituted systems and have no evidence showing whether or not our purified cytochrome P-450 has a function to hydroxylate *trans*-cinnamate. The purified form of cytochrome P-450 might not be specific only for *trans*-cinnamate but may also be present for other unknown substrates existing in limited tissues including tulip bulbs, because the *trans*-cinnamate 4-monooxygenase activity in tulip bulbs is quite low as compared with potato tubers, avocado mesocarps, and Jerusalem artichoke tubers (Table II). It is indicated that there is a heterogeneity of immunochemical properties of cytochrome P-450 proteins among various plant species; however, there has been no evidence to support immunochemically the presence of multiple forms of cytochrome P-450 from a single source of plant tissue.

In conclusion, the mechanism of cytochrome P-450-catalyzed reactions in plants has not been characterized nearly as thoroughly as the hepatic microsomal enzymes. The optical and magnetic characteristics of the plant cytochrome P-450 preparations closely resemble those of hepatic microsomes (45, 46). NADPH is a major source of electrons for the reduction of cytochrome P-450 in plants as in liver microsomes. An NADH-cytochrome c reductase and cytochrome b_5 can be also detected in plant microsomes and their participation in plant cytochrome P-450-dependent monooxygenase is unclear. No iron-sulphur proteins such as those found in mitochondrial and bacterial cytochrome P-450 electron-transport chains could be detected in the plant microsomes analyzed (46).

The plant cytochrome P-450 systems may be characterized by a high degree of substrate specificity (14, 24, 52, 53). In animal cells, especially in the liver, the microsomal cytochrome P-450 metabolizes a variety of xenobiotics with various chemical structures. Low substrate specificity of liver cytochrome P-450 is suitable for detoxication of a number of xenobiotics. Reconstituted monooxygenase with a highly purified form of cytochrome P-450 still shows relatively broad substrate specificity in animals (26, 30), although the presence of specific-forms for endogenous compounds, such as cholesterol metabolite (36) and prostaglandin (42) have been reported recently from animal sources. In general, the plant cytochrome P-450 systems may have a much narrower specificity for substrates than is found in the cytochrome P-450 species from liver. It is unknown whether a system equivalent to the drug-induced hepatic monooxygenase having a broad specificity is present in higher plants.

Metabolism of Environmental Chemicals by Higher Plants

It is important to know the transition and ultimate fate of environmental mutagens, both in amount and composition, in or on plants. This information is useful not only to elucidate their mode of action, but also to provide a basis for regulatory considerations.

Polycyclic aromatic hydrocarbon levels in soil and water affect human exposure through contaminated food and drinking water supplies. Environmental contaminants elevate the polycyclic aromatic hydrocarbon content of vegetation (3). Grain samples taken from industrial districts contain higher polycyclic aromatic hydrocarbon levels than samples from non-industrial areas, thus the setting and impaction of atmospheric aerosol may contaminate plants. Leafy plants, such as kale, spinach, and tobacco are found to contain high levels of benzo[a]pyrene but only a small portion is removable by washing (3).

An analysis, for example, of several common food items (fish, meat, field crops, and spices) sold in Nigerian markets has shown the presence of i) benzo[a]pyrene and benz[a]anthracene in fish and meat samples and ii) aflatoxin in crops and spices (12). These contaminations of the human diet could have a significant association with the relatively high incidence of human liver cancer in tropical African countries such as Nigeria.

The activation of chemicals (especially pesticides) into mutagens by green plants, noted by Plewa and Gentile (39), may be hazardous to the public health because of their widespread use in agriculture and the current lack of information about metabolic pathways. In vivo and in vitro plant assays have been reviewed by the same authors (40), and they pointed out that a class of plant promutagens distinct from mammalian promutagens may exist. Although plants can activate promutagenic chemicals into mutagens, some chemical mutagens can be detoxified by plant tissues. Conversion of agricultural chemicals into mutagens poses possible risks to public health and this problem must be studied further.

As a model system, we have examined the possible activation of either benzo[a]pyrene or aflatoxin B_1 by microsomes or S-9 fractions from Jerusalem artichoke tubers (18) or tulip bulbs (19). In these studies, the use of S-9 preparations from these higher plants, instead of rat liver, successfully induced back-mutation of Salmonella TA98. However, we noticed that the use of S-9 fraction from plant sources for examining the general environmental mutagens in the Ames' test had apparent limitations when compared with that of rat liver after Aroclor-treatment. A reproducible number of revertant colonies could be obtained only with relatively potent mutagens such as aflatoxin B1 due to the low levels of microsomal cytochrome P-450 and also the limited number of cytochrome P-450 types with narrow substrate specificity in the S-9 of plant sources. Furthermore, other factors specific for plant cells such as polyphenolic compounds might interfere with the metabolic activation of promutagens in S-9. So far, we have obtained no microsomal cytochrome P-450 equivalent to the hepatic drug-metabolizing system from plant sources.

Metabolites of benzo[a]pyrene with microsomes from cell suspension cultures of parsley (Petroselinum hortense Hoffm.), soybean (Glycine max. L.) (58), and Jerusalem artichoke tubers and tulip bulbs (23) have been analyzed with high performance liquid chromatography. The metabolites of benzo[a]pyrene by plant microsomes were mainly benzo[a]pyrene quinones and benzo[a]pyrene phenols, but few benzo[a]pyrene diols could be detected, although some polar components were found with tulips (23). Benzo[a]pyrene, added to the nutrient solutions of cell cultures of *Chenopodium rubrum* (goosefoot), was reported to be metabolized to oxygenated derivatives and some of these are linked to proteins or nucleic acids (16).

Filamentous fungus, *Cunninghamella elegans*, oxidized benzo[a]pyrene to several metabolic products, such as *trans*-9,10-dihydroxy-9,10-dihydrobenzo[a]pyrene, *trans*-7,8-dihydroxy-7,8-dihydrobenzo[a]pyrene, 3-hydroxy-benzo[a]pyrene *etc.*, although fungus is not a higher plant. However, it is interesting that benzo[a]pyrene is metabolized by a filamentous fungus in a manner remarkably similar to that observed in higher organisms (9).

It is still uncertain whether or not microsomal cytochrome P-450 plays a major role in the plant activation system. An *in vitro* reconstitution system of plant monooxygenase should be established to evaluate the role of microsomal cytochrome P-450 in the activation systems of higher plants.

Acknowledgments

The author is greatly indebted to Drs. Y. Karasaki, M. Obara, K. Ikeuchi, and K. Nakashima for their invaluable cooperation. This work was supported in part by Grants-in-Aid for Cancer Research and Environmental Science (Human Health Effects) from the Ministry of Education, Science and Culture, Japan.

REFERENCES

1. Adele, P., Reichhart, D., Salaün, J. P., Benveniste, I., and Durst, F. Induction of cytochrome P-450 and monooxygenase activity by 2,4-dichlorophenoxyacetic acid in higher plant tissue. *Plant. Sci. Lett.*, **22**, 39–46 (1981).
2. Attridge, T. H. and Smith, H. A phytochrome-mediated increase in the level of phenylalanine ammonia-lyase activity in the terminal buds of *Pisum sativum*. *Biochim. Biophys. Acta*, **148**, 805–807 (1967).
3. Baum, E. J. Occurrence and surveillance of polycyclic aromatic hydrocarbons. *In* "Polycyclic Hydrocarbons and Cancer," ed. H. V. Gelboin and P. O. Ts'o, Vol. 1, pp. 45–70 (1978). Academic Press, New York.
4. Benveniste, I., Salaün, J. P., and Durst, F. Wounding-induced cinnamic acid hydroxylase in Jerusalem Artichoke tuber. *Phytochemistry*, **16**, 69–73 (1977).
5. Benveniste, I., Salaün, J. P., and Durst, F. Phytochrome-mediated regulation of a monooxygenase hydroxylating cinnamic acid in etiolated pea seedlings. *Phytochemistry*, **17**, 359–363 (1978).
6. Benveniste, I., Gabriac, B., Fonne, R., Reichhart, D., Salaün, J. P., Simon, A., and Durst, F. Higher plant cytochrome P-450: microsomal electron transport and xenobiotics oxidation. *In* "Cytochrome P-450, Biochemistry, Biophysics and Environmental Implications," ed. E. Hietanen, M. Laitinen, and O. Hänninen, pp. 201–208 (1982). Elsevier Biomed. Press, Amsterdam.
7. Billett, E. E. and Smith, H. Control of phenylalanine ammonia lyase and cinnamic acid 4-hydroxylase in gherkin tissues. *Phytochemistry*, **19**, 1035–1041 (1980).
8. Casida, J. E. and Lykken, L. Metabolism of organic pesticide chemicals in higher plants. *Annu. Rev. Plant Physiol.*, **20**, 607–636 (1969).
9. Cerniglia, C. E. and Gibson, D. Oxidation of benzo(a)pyrene by the filamentous fungus

Cunninghamella elegans. J. Biol. Chem., **254**, 12174–12180 (1979).

10. Constantin, M. J. and Owens, E. T. Introduction and perspectives of plant genetic and cytogenetic assays: a report of the U. S. Environmental Protection Agency Gene-Tox Program. *Mut. Res.*, **99**, 1–12 (1982).

11. Dennis, D. R. and West, C. A. The conversion of (−)-kaurene to (−)-kauren-19-oic acid in endosperm of *Echinocystis macrocarpus* Greene. *J. Biol. Chem.*, **242**, 3293–3300 (1967).

12. Emerole, G. O., Uwaifo, A. O., Thabrew, M. I., and Bababunmi, E. A. The presence of aflatoxin and some polycyclic aromatic hydrocarbons in human foods. *Cancer Lett.*, **15**, 123–129 (1982).

13. Frear, D. S., Swanson, H. R., and Tanaka, F. S. N-demethylation of substituted 3-(phenyl)-1-methylureas: isolation and characterization of a microsomal mixed function oxidase from cotton. *Phytochemistry*, **8**, 2157–2169 (1969).

14. Gillard, D. F. and Walson, D. C. Abscisic acid metabolism by a cell-free preparation from *Echinocystis lobata* liquid endosperm. *Plant Physiol.*, **58**, 790–795 (1976).

15. Hahlbrock, K., Ebel, J., Ortmann, R., Sutter, A., Wellmann, E., and Grisebach, H. Regulation of enzyme activities related to the biosynthesis flavone glycosides in cell suspension cultures of parseley (*Petroselimun hortense*). *Biochim. Biophys. Acta*, **244**, 7–15 (1971).

16. Harms, H. Benzo(a)pyrene metabolites formed by plant cells. *Z. Naturforsch.*, **32c**, 321–326 (1977).

17. Hasson, D. P. and West, C. A. Properties of the system for the mixed function oxidation of kaurene and kaurene derivatives in microsomes of the immature seed of *Marah macrocarpus* (electron transfer components). *Plant Physiol.*, **58**, 479–484 (1976).

18. Higashi, K., Nakashima, K., Karasaki, Y., Fukunaga, M., and Mizuguchi, Y. Activation of benzo(a)pyrene by microsomes of higher plant tissues and their mutagenicity. *Biochem. Int.*, **2**, 373–380 (1981).

19. Higashi, K., Ikeuchi, K., and Karasaki, Y. Use of metabolic activation systems of tulip bulbs in the Ames test for environmental mutagens. *Bull. Environ. Contam. Toxicol.*, **29**, 505–510 (1982).

20. Higashi, K., Ikeuchi, K., Karasaki, Y., and Obara, M. Isolation of immunochemically distinct form of cytochrome P-450 from microsomes of tulip bulbs. *Biochem. Biophys. Res. Commun.*, **115**, 46–52 (1983).

21. Hill, A. C. and Rhodes, M.J.C. The properties of cinnamic acid 4-hydroxylase of aged swede root disks. *Phytochemistry*, **14**, 2387–2391 (1975).

22. Kahl, G. Metabolism in plant storage tissue slices. *Bot. Rev.*, **40**, 263–314 (1974).

23. Karasaki, Y. and Higashi, K. Metabolites of benzo(a)pyrene by microsomes of higher plants. *J. Univ. Occup. Environ. Health*, **4**, 417–424 (1982).

24. Karasaki, Y., Ikeuchi, K., and Higashi, K. Highly variable distributions of *trans*-cinnamate 4-monooxygenase in a variety of plant tissues. *J. Univ. Occup. Environ. Health*, **5**, 329–335 (1983).

25. Kolattukudy, P. E. and Walton, T. J. Structure and biosynthesis of the hydroxy fatty acids of cutin in *Vicia faba* leaves. *Biochemistry*, **11**, 1897–1907 (1972).

26. Koop, D. R., Persson, A. V., and Coon, M. J. Properties of electrophoretical homogeneous constitutive forms of liver microsomal cytochrome P-450. *J. Biol. Chem.*, **256**, 10704–10711 (1981).

27. Laemmli, U. K. Cleavage of structural proteins during the assembly of the head of bacteriophage T_4. *Nature*, **227**, 680–685 (1970).

28. Loomis, W. D. Overcoming problems of phenolics and quinones in the isolation of plant enzymes and organelles. *Methods Enzymol.*, **31**, 528–544 (1974).

29. Lord, J. M., Kagawa, T., Moore, T. S., and Beevers, H. Endoplasmic reticulum as the

site of lecithin formation in castor bean endosperm. *J. Cell Biol.*, **57**, 659–667 (1973).

30. Lu, A.Y.H. and West, S. B. Reconstituted mammalian mixed-function oxidase; requirements, specificities and other properties. *Pharmacol. Ther.*, **2**. 337–358 (1978).

31. Madyastha, K. M., Meehan, T. D., and Coscia, C. J. Characterization of a cytochrome P-450 dependent monoterpene hydroxylase from the higher plant *Vinca rosea*. *Biochemistry*, **15**, 1079–1102 (1976).

32. Madyastha, K. M., Ridgway, J. E., Dwyer, J. G., and Coscia, C. J. Subcellular localization of a cytochrome P-450-dependent monooxygenase in vesicles of the higher plant *Catharanthus roseus*. *J. Cell Biol.*, **72**, 302–313 (1977).

33. Markham, A., Hartman, G. C., and Parke, D. V. Spectral evidence for the presence of cytochrome P-450 in microsomal fractions obtained from some higher plants. *Biochem. J.*, **130**, 90 (1972).

34. Mathews, J. M. and Ortiz, R. Autocatalytic inactivation of plant cytochrome P-450 enzymes: Selective inactivation of cinnamic acid 4-hydroxylase from *Helianthus tuberosus* by 1-aminobenzotriazole. *Arch. Biochem. Biophys.*, **216**, 522–529 (1982).

35. Meehan, T. D. and Coscia, C. J. Hydroxylation of geraniol and nerol by a monooxygenase from *Vinca rosea*. *Biochem. Biophys. Res. Commun.*, **53**, 1043–1048 (1973).

36. Murakami, K., Okuda, Y., and Okuda, K. Purification and characterization of 7α-hydroxy-4-cholesten-3-one-12α-monooxygenase. *J. Biol. Chem.*, **257**, 8030–8035 (1982).

37. Murphy, P. J. and West, C. A. The role of mixed function oxidases in kaurene metabolism in *Echinocystis macrocarpa* Greene endosperm. *Arch. Biochem. Biophys.*, **113**, 395–407 (1969).

38. Ortiz, P. R. and Mico, B. A. Destruction of cytochrome P-450 by ethylene and other olefins. *Mol. Pharmacol.*, **18**, 128–135 (1980).

39. Plewa, M. J. and Gentile, J. M. Mutagenicity of atrazine: a maize-microbe bioassay. *Mut. Res.*, **38**, 287–292 (1976).

40. Plewa, M. J. and Gentile, J. M. The activation of chemicals into mutagens by green plants. *In* "Chemical Mutagens: Principles and Methods for Their Detection," ed. F. J. Serres and A. Hollaender, pp. 401–420 (1982). Plenum, New York.

41. Potts, J.R.M., Weklych, R., and Conn, E. E. The 4-hydroxylation of cinnamic acid by sorghum microsomes and the requirement for cytochrome P-450. *J. Biol. Chem.*, **249**, 5019–5026 (1974).

42. Powell, W. S. ω-Oxidation of prostaglandins by lung and liver microsomes. *J. Biol. Chem.*, **253**, 5019–5026 (1978).

43. Reichhart, D., Salaün, J.-P., Benveniste, I., and Durst, F. Induction by manganese, ethanol, phenobarbital, and herbicides of microsomal cytochrome P-450 in higher plant tissues. *Arch. Biochem. Biophys.*, **196**, 301–303 (1979).

44. Reichhart, D., Salaün, J.-P., Benveniste, I., and Durst, F. Time course of induction of cytochrome P-450, NADPH-cytochrome *c* reductase, and cinnamic acid hydroxylase by phenobarbital, ethanol, herbicides and manganese in higher plant microsomes. *Plant Physiol.*, **66**, 600–604 (1980).

45. Rich, P. R. and Bendall, D. S. Cytochrome components of plant microsomes. *Eur. J. Biochem.*, **55**, 333–341 (1975).

46. Rich, P. R., Cammack, R., and Bendall, D. S. Electron paramagnetic resonance studies of cytochrome P-450 in plant microsomes. *Eur. J. Biochem.*, **59**, 281–286 (1975).

47. Rich, P. R. and Lamb, C. J. Biophysical and enzymological studies upon the interaction of *trans*-cinnamic acid with higher plant microsomal cytochrome P-450. *Eur. J. Biochem.*, **72**, 353–360 (1977).

48. Russell, D. W. and Conn, E. E. The cinnamic acid-4-hydroxylase of pea seedlings. *Arch. Biochem. Biophys.*, **122**, 256–258 (1967).

49. Russell, D. W. The metabolism of aromatic compounds in higher plants X. properties of the cinnamic acid 4-hydroxylase of pea seedlings and some aspects of its metabolic and developmental control. *J. Biol. Chem.*, **246**, 3870–3878 (1971).

50. Saito, T. and Strobel, H. W. Purification to homogeneity and characterization of a form of cytochrome P-450 with high specificity for benzo(a)pyrene from β-naphthoflavone-pretreated rat liver microsomes. *J. Biol. Chem.*, **256**, 984–988 (1981).

51. Salaün J. P., Benveniste, I., Reichhart, D., and Durst, F. A microsomal (cytochrome P-450)-linked lauric-acid-monooxygenase from aged Jerusalem-artichoke-tuber tissues. *Eur. J. Biochem.*, **90**, 155–159 (1978).

52. Salaün, J-P., Benveniste, I., Feyereisen, R., and Durst, F. Product specificity and regulation of two laurate hydroxylases in higher plants. *In* "Microsomes, Drug Oxidations, and Chemical Carcinogenesis," ed. M. J. Coon *et al.*, pp. 721–724 (1980). Academic Press, New York.

53. Salaün, J. P., Benveniste, I., Reichhart, D., and Durst, F. Induction and specificity of a (cytochrome P-450)-dependent laurate in-chain-hydroxylase from higher plant microsomes. *Eur. J. Biochem.*, **119**, 651–655 (1981).

54. Soliday, C. L. and Kolattukudy, P. E. Biosynthesis of cutin ω-hydroxylation of fatty acids by a microsomal preparation from germinating *Vicia faba*. *Plant Physiol.*, **59**, 1116–1121 (1977).

55. Soliday, C. L. and Kolattukudy, P. E. Midchain hydroxylation of 16-hydroxypalmitic acid by the endoplasmic reticulum fraction from germinating *Vicia faba*. *Arch Biochem. Biophys.*, **188**, 338–347 (1978).

56. Steveninck, R. The "washing" of "aging" phenomenon in plant tissues. *Annu. Rev. Plant Physiol.*, **26**, 237–258 (1975).

57. Tanaka, F. S., Swanson, H. R., and Frear, D. S. Mechanism of oxidative N-demethylation by cotton microsomes. *Phytochemistry*, **11**, 2709–2715 (1972).

58. Trenck, Th.v.d. and Sandermann, H., Jr. Oxygenation of benzo(a)pyrene by plant microsomal fractions. *FEBS Lett.*, **119**, 227–231 (1980).

59. Young, O. and Beevers, H. Mixed function oxidases from germinating castor bean endosperm. *Phytochemistry*, **15**, 379–385 (1976).

60. West, C. A. Hydroxylases, monooxygenases, and cytochrome P-450. *In* "The Biochemistry of Plants," ed. P. K. Stumph and E. E. Conn, Vol. 2, pp. 317–364 (1980). Academic Press, New York.

61. Whightman, R. and Setterfield, G. Cytological responses in Jerusalem artichoke tuber slices during aging and subsequent auxin treatment. *In* "Physiology and Biochemistry of Plant Growth," ed. L. C. Fowke and G. Setterfield, pp. 581–602 (1968). Runge Press, Ottawa.

ACTIVATION OF CARCINOGENIC COMPOUNDS BY CYTOCHROME P-450

METABOLIC ACTIVATION OF CHEMICAL CARCINOGENS BY TWO MOLECULAR SPECIES OF CYTOCHROME P-450

Yusaku TAGASHIRA, Hiromichi YONEKAWA, Junko WATANABE, Eiichi HARA, Jun-ichi HAYASHI, Osamu GOTOH, and Kaname KAWAJIRI

Department of Biochemistry, Saitama Cancer Center Research Institute*

We investigated the roles of two major forms of rat liver microsomal cytochrome P-450, phenobarbital (PB)-P-450 and methylcholanthrene (MC)-P-448, in the metabolic activation process of various chemical carcinogens such as aromatic hydrocarbons, aromatic amines, azo dyes, and nitrosocompounds. To estimate the contributions of the two forms of cytochrome P-450, we adopted an inhibition assay system. We prepared antibodies to the individual forms of cytochrome P-450 and to NADPH-cytochrome P-450 reductase; these antibodies were used as specific inhibitors of mutagenic activation in the Ames' assay system. Since the microsomes prepared from polychlorinated biphenyls (PCB)-treated rats contained nearly equal amounts of two major forms of cytochrome P-450, each comprising about 40% of total cytochrome P-450, the contributions of cytochrome of P-450 forms to mutagenic activation were easily estimated from the rates of inhibition by the antibodies. We then found that the two major forms of cytochrome P-450 contribute most to the metabolic activation of all carcinogens tested. Their relative contributions varied greatly depending on the carcinogens. Our finding was also supported by two other experiments: the binding of carcinogens to nuclear DNA was completely inhibited by the antibodies; the formation of metabolites of carcinogens was also markedly inhibited by the antibodies.

By immunoprecipitation methods, we then determined the contents of the two forms of cytochrome P-450 in the liver microsomes of rats which had been administered by a single dose of carcinogen, and found that the induction differed. On the basis of the specific activities and contents of the two cytochrome P-450 forms, we could estimate their contributions to the metabolic activation of carcinogens in microsomes. Our estimation agreed well with experimental observation of the Ames' test with S-9 fraction. This result suggests that at least two factors must be considered to explain metabolic activation of carcinogens *in vivo*: (a) the specific activity of cytochrome P-450 forms to the formation of active metabolites, and (b) the contents of cytochrome P-450 forms depending on carcinogens.

Most chemical carcinogens and mutagens require metabolic activation before they exert their deleterious effects on an organism (*6, 18*). In this activation process, the first step is usually carried out by the mixed function oxidase system of microsomes

---

* Komuro 818, Ina-machi, Kitaadachi-gun, Saitama 362, Japan (田頭勇作, 米川博通, 渡辺潤子, 原栄一, 林 純一, 後藤 修, 川尻 要).

(6, 18). This system is composed of NADPH-cytochrome P-450 reductase and cytochrome P-450. Recently evidence has accumulated for the existence of multiple forms
of cytochrome P-450 (15, 26). These forms have different substrate specificities and
participate in various pathways of the activation and detoxification of numerous xenobiotics in liver cells (15, 26).

However, little has been known about the contribution of each form of cytochrome
P-450 to the activation of carcinogens. Two methods are then useful to study the roles
of specific forms of cytochrome P-450 in the metabolic activation of carcinogens; one
is based on the reconstituted systems of microsomal monooxygenase using purified
cytochrome P-450 preparations (2, 20, 31–34), and the other is inhibition tests using
specific antibodies (3, 4, 7, 11–14, 35). The former method is very useful in assessing
the participation of each cytochrome P-450 form in metabolic activation. However,
the information obtained by reconstituted systems seems unsuited to the evaluation of
relative importance of each cytochrome P-450 species in the activation of carcinogens
in intact microsomes, since various forms of this cytochrome coexist in the microsomal
membrane (29, 30). On the other hand, the relative importance of each cytochrome
P-450 species in intact systems can be evaluated by the inhibition tests, since each of
the specific antibodies selectively inhibits the reaction catalyzed by a particular form
of cytochrome P-450 which raises the antibody (13). The most efficient assay system,
then, is by this inhibition test in combination with the Ames' mutation test. Since a
good correlation between carcinogenicity and mutagenicity has been established for
various chemical compounds (16, 17, 19), the bacterial mutation system enabled us
to estimate the relative importance of a specific form of cytochrome P-450 in carcinogenesis. In this article, we describe our experimental results on the role of different
forms of cytochrome P-450 in the metabolic activation of carcinogens and discuss their
significance in mutagenesis and carcinogenesis *in vivo*.

Preparation of Antibodies to Microsomal Electron Transport Components

Two respective types of cytochrome P-450, PB-P-450 and MC-P-448, which are
major components of rat liver microsomes pretreated with phenobarbital (PB) and

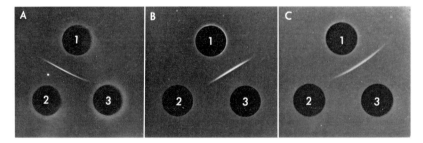

FIG. 1.   Ouchterlony immunodiffusion test of the antibodies. A: well 1 contained antibody to PB-P-450. Wells 2 and 3 contained partially purified PB-P-450
and MC-P-448, respectively. B: well 1 contained antibody to MC-P-448. Wells
2 and 3 were the same as for A. C: well 1 contained antibody to NADPH-cytochrome P-450 reductase. Wells 2 and 3 contained buffer and partially purified
NADPH-cytochrome P-450 reductase, respectively.

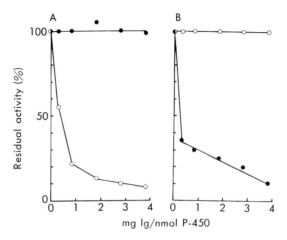

Fig. 2. Effects of antibodies on microsomal drug oxidations. Liver microsomes of rats treated with PCB were preincubated with antibodies at 25°C for 10 min. Activities in the presence of anti-PB-P-450 Ig (●) or anti-MC-P-448 IG (○) are shown as the percentages of activities assayed with control Ig. A: BP hydroxylation. B: benzphetamine N-demethylation.

3-methylcholanthrene (MC), were isolated (5) together with NADPH-cytochrome P-450 reductase (F_{PT}) (22). Antibodies against these three purified preparations were prepared from rabbit antisera (13, 21). The specificity of these antibodies was tested by Ouchterlony double-diffusion analysis and also by their inhibition effects on microsomal drug oxidation activities. It was confirmed that each antibody selectively reacts with the corresponding antigen in Fig. 1. Furthermore, benzo[a]pyrene hydroxylation and benzophetamine N-demethylation were completely inhibited by anti-MC-P-448 immunoglobulin (Ig) and anti-PB-P-450 Ig, respectively, when these antibodies were added to the liver microsomes of polychlorynated biphenyls (PCB)-treated rats (Fig. 2). These results are compatible with the substrate specificities of two forms of cytochrome P-450 examined in a reconstituted system of monooxygenase. Using those antibodies, we can thus identify specific forms of cytochrome P-450 involved in the metabolic activation of carcinogens.

Specific Forms of Cytochrome P-450 Involved in Mutagenesis

Table I shows the contents of PB-P-450 and MC-P-448 in microsomes from untreated and PCB-treated rat livers, determined by the immunoprecipitation method (5). The total amount of cytochrome P-450 in PCB-treated microsomes was about three times larger than that in untreated microsomes. The contents of PB-P-450 and MC-P-448 in PCB-treated microsomes were nearly equal, accounting for over 80% of the total cytochrome P-450, while they accounted for only 20% of the total in untreated microsomes. PCB-treated microsomes of the S-9 fraction, which are usually used in the Ames tests, are thus found to identify the specific forms of cytochrome P-450 involved in mutagenesis by carcinogens.

Figure 3 demonstrates this by way of example. The mutagenic activity of Trp-P-1, a potent mutagen, was inhibited 92 and 89% by antibodies to F_{PT} and to MC-P-448,

Y. TAGASHIRA ET AL.

TABLE I. Contents of PB-P-450 and MC-P-448 in Microsomes from
Uninduced and PCB-induced Rat Livers

	Total P-450 (μg/mg[a]) (%)	PB-P-450 (μg/mg) (%)	MC-P-448 (μg/mg) (%)
Uninduced microsomes	45.0 (100)	6.0 (13)	4.0 (9)
PCB-induced microsomes	166.0 (100)	75.0 (45)	60.0 (36)

[a] μg per mg of microsomal protein.

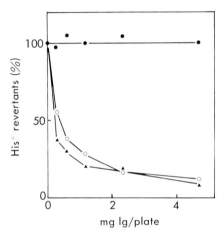

FIG. 3. Effects of antibodies on the mutagenic activities of Trp-P-1. The His[+]
revertants in the presence of anti-PB-P-450 Ig (●), anti-MC-P-448 Ig (○), or
anti-F_{PT} Ig (▲) are shown as the percentages of the His[+] revertants assayed with
control Ig. Strain TA 98 was used in this experiment.

respectively, whereas the antibody to PB-P-450 did not inhibit this activity. NADPH-
cytochrome P-450 reductase exists as a single form and mediates the electron transfer
from NADPH to all forms of cytochrome P-450 in microsomal membranes. Thus, the
rate of inhibition by anti-F_{PT}-Ig means the total activity mediated by various forms
of cytochrome P-450, even if different molecular species of the cytochrome participate
in the mutagenic activation of each carcinogen. Accordingly, it was concluded that the
mutagenic activation of Trp-P-1 almost exclusively depends on MC-P-448.

Figure 4 summarizes the results obtained from similar experiments on some re-
presentative carcinogens such as aromatic hydrocarbons, aromatic amines, azo dyes,
and nitroso compounds. The vertical and horizontal axes indicate the dependency of
mutagenic activation on PB-P-450 and MC-P-448, respectively. From this diagram,
two conclusions can be drawn. First, the mutagenic activations of all carcinogens
tested primarily depend on PB-P-450 and MC-P-448, because all the points in the
diagram fall around the cross-diagonal line. Since the sum of the inhibition rates of
these two cytochrome P-450 forms is nearly 100% for all the carcinogens tested, the
initial step in their activation is most likely participated in by the NADPH-dependent
electron transport system. Second, various carcinogens can be classified into four
groups according to the dependency of their activation on the two forms of cytochrome
P-450 (*13, 14*): (a) Activated selectively by MC-P-448 (benzo[a]pyren(BP), 7,12-

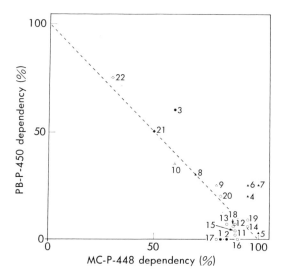

Fɪɢ. 4. Dependency of metabolic activation of chemical carcinogens on two forms of cytochrome P-450. 1, BP; 2, DMBA; 3, MC; 4, DAB; 5, 3'-MeDAB; 6, MAB; 7, 3'-MeMAB; 8, OAT; 9, 2-NA; 10, 2-AAF; 11, Trp-P-1; 12, Trp-P-2; 13, Glu-P-1; 14, Glu-P-2; 15, IQ; 16, MeIQ; 17, AαC; 18, MeAαC; 19, 3-Ac-Trp-P-1; 20, Lys-P-1; 21, DMN; 22, AFB$_1$.

dimethylbenzanthracene (DMBA), p-dimethylaminoazobenzene (DAB), Trp-P-1, *etc.*), (b) activated predominantly by MC-P-448 (2-naphthylamine (2-NA), 2-acetylamino-fluorene (2-AAF), *etc.*), (c) activated equally by both MC-P-448 and PB-P-450 (N-nitrosodimethylamine (DMN), 3-MC), and (d) activated predominantly by PB-P-450 (aflatoxin B$_1$ (AFB$_1$)). It is then remarkable that the majority of carcinogens belong to groups (a) and (b).

Mutation appears as a result of the complex processes of successive reactions including such important ones as the formation of proximate forms of carcinogens and the binding of carcinogens to DNA. Consequently, the two antibodies must inhibit these two important reactions by degrees similar to those obtained by the mutation test (see Fig. 4).

The formation of 7,8-diol BP, a proximate form of BP, was completely inhibited by the antibody to MC-P-448 but hardly inhibited by that to PB-P-450, when we analyzed its metabolites by high pressure liquid chromatography (*4*). N-OH-AAF, a proximate form of 2-AAF, was also inhibited in its formation about 70 and 30% by the antibodies to MC-P-448 and to PB-P-450, respectively (*3*). These inhibition rates are the same as those obtained in the mutation tests.

Furthermore, we found that the inhibition of the DNA-binding of BP, 2-AAF, and AFB$_1$ by the antibodies well corresponded to the results in the mutation tests (*12*).

Mutagenic Activation in Untreated Microsomes

PB-P-450 and MC-P-448 each comprise only about 10% of the cytochrome P-450 in the untreated microsomes, as shown in Table I. So the remaining about 80% of the total must be composed of other forms of cytochrome P-450. Accordingly, the S-9

Y. TAGASHIRA ET AL.

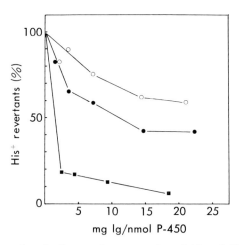

FIG. 5. Effects of antibodies on the mutagenic activities of AFB_1 mediated by
the liver S-9 fraction of untreated rats. The His^+ revertants in the presence of
anti-PB-P-450 Ig (●), anti-MC-P-448 Ig (○), or anti-F_{PT} Ig (▲) are shown as
percentages of the His^+ revertants assayed with control Ig.

fraction of untreated rats is used to determine the participation of other forms of cytochrome P-450 on the mutagenic activation of chemical carcinogens, although the overall
mutagenicity of carcinogens activated by untreated S-9 fraction is distinctively lower
than that by PCB-treated S-9. Figure 5 shows the inhibition effects of the antibodies
to microsomal F_{PT}, PB-P-450 and MC-P-448 on the mutagenicities of AFB_1. The
inhibition rates by the antibodies to PB-P-450 and MC-P-448 were 60 and 40%,
respectively, and their sum was almost equal to the inhibition by the antibody to F_{PT}.
A similar profile was also obtained for Trp-P-2 and 2-AAF, which have relatively
high mutagenic activities in untreated S-9 fraction (11). Thus, it is concluded that
PB-P-450 and MC-P-448, which compose a minor part of the total cytochrome P-450
in untreated S-9 fraction, mainly participate in the microsomal activation of these
carcinogens. The low mutagenic activity of carcinogens in untreated S-9 is then ascribed
to the low concentrations of PB-P-450 and MC-P-448 in the liver microsomes of
untreated rats (11).

Induction of Cytochrome P-450 by Carcinogens

3-Methylcholanthrene is a potent specific inducer of MC-P-448. Some other
carcinogens are also known to act as inducers of certain forms of P-450 (15, 26). Accordingly, the inducibility of a carcinogen to the specific forms of P-450, which is
responsible for its activation, is an important factor for its overall carcinogenic potency
in vivo (11). To evaluate this effect, we measured the contents of two forms of P-450,
PB-P-450 and MC-P-448, after the administration of single doses of various carcinogens
to rats. Mutagenicity of these carcinogens was also tested with the S-9 fraction prepared
in the same time course as the above measurement after the administration.

In the experiments shown in Fig. 6A, a single dose of O-aminoazotoluene (OAT)
was given to rats at time zero, and the contents of total cytochrome P-450, PB-P-450
and MC-P-448 in microsomes were measured at various time points. Total cytochrome

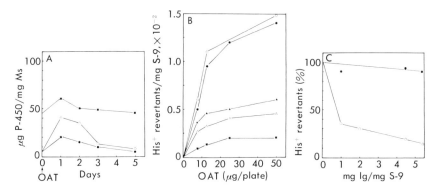

FIG. 6. A: changes in the contents of PB-P-450 and MC-P-448 in microsomes of OAT-treated rats. OAT was injected i.p. into rats, and the total content of cytochrome P-450 (■), PB-P-450 (●), and MC-P-448 (○) were assayed at various time points. B: changes in the mutagenic activity of OAT in the liver S-9 fraction after a single dose of OAT to rats. After the administration of OAT, S-9 fraction was prepared at various time points. A fixed amount of S-9 fraction was incubated with various amounts of OAT as indicated in the figure, and the strain TA 98 His$^+$ revertants were assayed at the following times after the injection of OAT. ■ S-9 fraction of uninduced rats; ○ 1 day; ● 2 days; ▲ 3 days; △ 5 days. C: effects of antibodies on the mutagenicity of OAT in the S-9 fraction of OAT-treated rats. S-9 fraction was prepared from OAT-treated rats 24 hr after the injection of OAT. OAT was incubated with the S-9 fraction in the presence of antibodies. ● anti-PB-P-450 Ig; ○ anti-MC-P-448 Ig.

P-450 increased only by about 30% at 24 hr after the administration of OAT, however, MC-P-448 and PB-P-450 respectively increased about 10 and 5 times. Figure 6B shows the time course of mutagenic activity of OAT in the S-9 fraction prepared from pretreated rats. The mutagenic activity of OAT reached a maximum of about seven times as high as that of untreated rats at 24–48 hr after the administration. Thus, a good correlation was found between the contents of the two forms of P-450 and the mutagenic activity throughout the time course of induction by OAT.

Figure 6C shows the effect of the antibodies against PB-P-450 and MC-P-448 on the mutagenic activity of OAT in S-9 fraction 24 hr after the administration. Anti-PB-P-450 Ig and anti-MC-P-448 Ig respectively inhibited the mutagenicity by 15 and 85%, giving a ratio of 3:17. The ratio of relative specific activities of PB-P-450 and MC-P-448 for mutagenicity of OAT was 3:7 (Fig. 4), while the ratio of their contents in the liver microsomes of OAT-induced rats was 1:2 (Fig. 6A). From these values, we can calculate the ratio of contributions of PB-P-450 and MC-P-448 to the activation of OAT as 3:14. This ratio well agrees with the observed value of 3:17, which was obtained with the specific antibodies and the S-9 fraction of OAT-induced rats.

Similar experiments on other carcinogens revealed that they may be classified into three groups according to their inducibility to PB-P-450 and MC-P-448: (a) those inducing both MC-P-448 and PB-P-450 (OAT), (b) inducing selectively MC-P-448 (BP, 3-MC), and (c) ineffective to the levels of both MC-P-448 and PB-P-450 (AFB$_1$) (11).

Therefore, both the substrate specificities and the contents of the two forms of cytochrome P-450 are important *in vivo* for the metabolic activation of carcinogens of groups (a) and (b), whereas the substrate specificity is the major factor for the activation of group (c).

DISCUSSION

There is increasing evidence that environmental chemicals, both man-made and natural, play an important role in causing human cancer (25, 27). The initial recognition of the importance of metabolic activation was achieved by Miller and Miller who reached the following general conclusions (18): (a) All chemical carcinogens which are not chemically reactive by themselves must be converted metabolically into reactive forms, (b) the activated metabolites are electrophilic reagents, and (c) these metabolites react with nucleophilic groups in cellular macromolecules to initiate carcinogenesis. Furthermore, they have discovered that these metabolic activations occur primarily through the microsomal monooxygenase system.

A simple test system which is useful for the survey of chemical carcinogens and mutagens has been developed by Ames and his coworkers during the last ten years (1). The test examines the mutagenicity of chemicals in a bacterial system and has proven to be about 90% accurate in detecting carcinogenicity. Since mutagenic activities of various chemical carcinogens tested were completely inhibited by the antibody to microsomal NADPH-cytochrome P-450 reductase (F_{PT}), the microsomal monooxygenase system occupies an essential part in the metabolic pathways of these carcinogens.

The monooxygenase of microsomes is a multi-enzyme system which is composed of F_{PT} and cytochrome P-450. Multiple forms of cytochrome P-450 are present, and some of them are inducible in different ways by the administration of chemical compounds including some carcinogens (15, 26). The content of each cytochrome P-450 and its molecular architecture, which was formed by the flavoprotein and different forms of P-450 in microsomal membrane, are uniquely determined and variable according to the induced state of animals (26). Thus, it is essential to determine what molecular forms of cytochrome P-450 participate in the metabolic activation of chemical carcinogens in intact microsomes (13).

We must consider at least two factors in evaluating the contribution of each form of cytochrome P-450 to the metabolic activation of carcinogens in microsomes (11): (a) The specific catalytic activity of cytochrome P-450 forms on carcinogens, and (b) the content of each cytochrome P-450 in microsomes of carcinogen-treated animals. We have disclosed the role of two major forms of cytochrome P-450, PB-P-450 and MC-P-448, in the mutagenesis of carcinogens. Using antibodies specific to respective cytochrome P-450 forms, the relative activity of each P-450 to various species of carcinogens was estimated by an inhibition test as shown in Fig. 4. We found that all the mutagenic activities by carcinogens were attributable to the two forms of cytochrome P-450, and that the contribution of each P-450 form to the activation differed among various carcinogens. We also found a good correlation between the increase of mutagenic activity and the contents of the two P-450 forms in microsomes by the administration of carcinogens to rats.

Our immunochemical determination of the contributions of PB-P-450 and MC-P-448 to the metabolic activation of carcinogens depended upon the specificity of the antibodies used. Recent studies by Levin and his coworkers on the multiple P-450 forms in rat liver microsomes (23, 24, 29, 30) have confirmed immunological cross-reactivity among some of them. P-450b, which was denoted as PB-P-450 in this paper, was immunologically identical with a minor form, P-450e (24). P-450c denoted as MC-P-448 by us showed partial immuno-cross-reactivity with another form, P-450d (23). In view of their observations, our preparation of anti-PB-P-450 Ig or anti-MC-P-448 Ig possibly recognizes some other molecular species of P-450. Thus, we are now trying to purify the antibody to MC-P-448 by an immunoadsorption method to remove the components which are cross-reacting with P-450d.

Recently, cDNA clone for P-450d (9, 10) and genomic clone for P-450c (28) were isolated. Comparison of the nucleotide sequences of cDNA and the gene revealed that the coding nucleotide sequences are composed of highly- and weakly-homologous blocks (8). This suggests that we can discriminate messenger RNA of P-450c from that of P-450d using specific fragments of cloned DNA sequences as hybridization probes. To understand the molecular mechanism of metabolic activation of carcinogens by cytochrome P-450, study at the gene level will be important in the future.

Acknowledgments

We wish to thank Dr. K. Nakachi (Department of Epidemiology, Saitama Cancer Center Research Institute) for his critical reading of the manuscript. This work was supported in part by a Grant-in-Aid for Cancer Research from the Ministry of Education Science and Culture of Japan.

REFERENCES

1. Ames, B. N., McCann, J., and Yamasaki, E. Methods for detecting carcinogens and mutagens with the *Salmonella*/mammalian-microsome mutagenicity test. *Mut. Res.*, **31**, 347–364 (1975).
2. Deutsch, J., Leutz, J. C., Yang, S. K., Gelboin, H. V., Chiang, Y. L., Vatsis, K. P., and Coon, M. J. Regio- and stereoselectivity of various forms of purified cytochrome P-450 in the metabolism of benzo(a)pyrene and (−)*trans*-7, 8-dihydroxy-7, 8-dihydrobenzo(a)-pyrene as shown by product formation and binding to DNA. *Proc. Natl. Acad. Sci. U. S.*, **74**, 3123–3127 (1978).
3. Hara, E., Kawajiri, K., Gotoh, O., and Tagashira, Y. Immunochemical study on the contributions of two molecular species of microsomal cytochrome P-450 to the metabolism of 2-acetylaminofluorene by rat liver microsomes. *Cancer Res.*, **41**, 253–257 (1981).
4. Hara, E., Kawajiri, K., and Tagashira, Y. Immunochemical study on the contributions of two molecular species of microsomal cytochrome P-450 to the metabolism of benzo(a)-pyrene by rat liver microsomes. *Cancer Res.*, **43**, 3604–3608 (1983).
5. Harada, N. and Omura, T. Selective induction of two different molecular species of cytochrome P-450 by phenobarbital and 3-methylcholanthrene. *J. Biochem.*, **89**, 237–248 (1981).
6. Heidelberger, C. Chemical carcinogenesis. *Annu. Rev. Biochem.*, **44**, 79–121 (1975).
7. Igarashi, S., Yonekawa, H., Kawajiri, K., Watanabe, J., Kimura, T., Kodama, M., Nagata, C., and Tagashira, Y. Participation of the microsomal electron transport system in mutagenic activation of 4-dimethylaminoazobenzene, 4-methyl-aminoazobenzene and their 3′-methyl-derivatives. *Biochem. Biophys. Res. Commun.*, **106**, 164–169 (1982).
8. Kawajiri, K., Gotoh, O., Sogawa, K., Tagashira, Y., Muramatsu, M., and Fujii-Kuri-

yama, Y. Coding nucleotide sequence of 3-methylcholanthrene-inducible cytochrome P-450d cDNA from rat liver. *Proc. Natl. Acad. Sci. U. S.*, **81**, 1649–1653 (1984).

9. Kawajiri, K., Gotoh, O., Tagashira, Y., Sogawa, K., Fuji-Kuriyama, Y. Titrations of mRNA for cytochrome P-450c and P-450d under drug-inductive conditions in rat livers by their specific probes of cloned DNAs. *J. Biol. Chem.*, **259**, 10145–10149 (1984).

10. Kawajiri, K., Sogawa, K., Gotoh, O., Tagashira, Y., Muramatsu, M., and Fujii-Kuriyama, Y. Molecular cloning of a complementary DNA to 3-methylcholanthrene-inducible cytochrome P-450 mRNA from rat liver. *J. Biochem.*, **94**, 1465–1473 (1983).

11. Kawajiri, K., Yonekawa, H., Gotoh, O., Watanabe, J., Igarashi, S., and Tagashira, Y. Contributions of two inducible forms of cytochrome P-450 in rat liver microsomes to the metabolic activation of various chemical carcinogens. *Cancer Res.*, **43**, 819–823 (1983).

12. Kawajiri, K., Yonekawa, H., Hara, E., and Tagashira, Y. Participation of two molecular species of cytochrome P-450 in the metabolic activation of carcinogens in the nuclei of rat liver. Proc. Jpn. Cancer. Assoc., The 40th Annual Meeting, pp. 80 (1981).

13. Kawajiri, K., Yonekawa, H., Harada, N., Noshiro, M., Omura, T., and Tagashira, Y. Immunochemical study on the role of different types of microsomal cytochrome P-450 in mutagenesis by chemical carcinogens. *Cancer Res.*, **40**, 1652–1657 (1980).

14. Kawajiri, K., Yonekawa, H., Watanabe, J., Igarashi, S., and Tagashira, Y. The role of two major types of microsomal cytochrome P-450 in the metabolic activation of chemical carcinogens. *In* "Microsomes, Drug Oxidations and Drug Toxicity," ed. R. Sato and R. Kato, pp. 535–536 (1982). Japan Sci. Soc. Press, Tokyo / Wiley-Interscience, New York.

15. Lu, A.H.Y. and West, S. B. Multiplicity of mammalian microsomal cytochromes P-450. *Pharmacol. Rev.*, **31**, 277–295 (1980).

16. McCann, J. and Ames, B. N. Detection of carcinogens as mutagens in the *Salmonella* / microsome test: assay of 300 chemicals: discussion. *Proc. Natl. Acad. Sci. U. S.*, **73**, 950–954 (1976).

17. McCann, J., Choi, E., Yamasaki, E., and Ames, B. N. Detection of carcinogens as mutagens in the *Salmonella* / microsomes test: assay of 300 chemicals. *Proc. Natl. Acad. Sci. U. S.*, **72**, 5135–5139 (1975).

18. Miller E. C. and Miller, J. A. Biochemical mechanism of chemical carcinogenesis. *In* "The Molecular Biology of Cancer," ed. H. Busch, pp. 377–402 (1974). Academic Press, New York.

19. Nagao, M., Sugimura, T., and Matsushima, T. Environmental mutagens and carcinogens. *Annu. Rev. Genet.*, **12**, 117–159 (1978).

20. Norman, R. L., Muller-Eberhand, U., and Johnson, E. F. The role of cytochrome P-450 forms in 2-aminoanthracene and benzo(a)pyrene mutagenesis. *Biochem. Biophys. Res. Commun.*, **89**, 195–201 (1979).

21. Noshiro, M. and Omura, T. Immunochemical Study on the electron pathway from NADH to cytochrome P-450 of liver microsomes. *J. Biochem.*, **83**, 61–77 (1978).

22. Omura, T. and Takesue, S. A new method for simultaneous purification of cytochrome b_5 and NADPH-cytochrome c reductase from rat liver microsomes. *J. Biochem.*, **67**, 249–257 (1970).

23. Reik, L. M., Levin, W., Ryan, D. E., and Thomas, P. E. Immunochemical relatedness of rat hepatic microsomal cytochromes P-450c and P-450d. *J. Biol. Chem.*, **257**, 3950–3957 (1982).

24. Ryan, D. E., Thomas, P. E., and Levin, W. Purification and characterization of a minor form of hepatic microsomal cytochrome P-450 from rats treated with polychlorinated biphenyls. *Arch. Biochem. Biophys.*, **216**, 272–288 (1982).

25. Sax, N. I. "Cancer Causing Chemicals," pp. 1–466 (1981). Van Nostrand Reinhold Company, New York.
26. Sato, R. and Omura, T. eds. "Cytochrome P-450," pp. 1–233 (1978). Kodansha, Tokyo/Academic Press, New York and London.
27. Sugimura, J., Nagao, M., Kawachi, T., Honda, M., Yahagi, J., Seino, Y., Sato, S., and Matsukura, N. Mutagen-carcinogens in foods, with special reference to highly mutagenic pyrolytic products in broiled foods. *In* "Origins of Human Cancer," ed. H. H. Hiatt, J. D. Watson, and J. A. Winsten, pp. 1561–1577 (1977). Cold Spring Harbor, New York.
28. Sogawa, K., Gotoh, O., Kawajiri, K., and Fujii-Kuriyama, Y. Distinct organization of methylcholanthrene- and phenobarbital-inducible cytochrome P-450 genes in the rat. *Proc. Natl. Acad. Sci. U. S.*, **81**, 5066–5070 (1984).
29. Thomas, P. E., Reik, L. M., Ryan, D. E., and Levin, W. Regulation of three forms of cytochrome P-450 and epoxide hydrolase in rat liver microsomes. *J. Biol. Chem.*, **256**, 1044–1052 (1981).
30. Thomas, P. E., Reik, L. M., Ryan, D. E., and Levin, W. Induction of two immunologically related rat liver cytochrome P-450 isozymes, cytochrome P-450c and P-450d, by structually diverse xenobiotics. *J. Biol. Chem.*, **258**, 4590–4598 (1983).
31. Wood, A. W., Chang, R. L., Levin, W., Thomas, P. E., Ryan, D., Stoming, T. A., Thakker, D. R., Jerina, D. M., and Conney, A. H. Metabolic activation of 3-methylcholanthrene and its metabolites to products mutagenic to bacterial and mammalian cells. *Cancer Res.*, **38**, 3398–3404 (1978).
32. Wood, A. W., Levin, W., Lu, A.Y.H., Yagi, H., Hernandez, U., Jerina, D. M., and Conney, A. H. Metabolism of benzo(a)pyrene and benzo(a)pyrene derivatives to mutagenic products by highly purified hepatic microsomal enzymes. *J. Biol. Chem.*, **251**, 4882–4890 (1976).
33. Wood, A. W., Levin, W., Thakker, D. R., Yagi, H., Chang, R. L., Ryan, D. E., Thomas, P. E., Dansette, P. M., Whittaker, N., Turuiman, S., Lehr, R. E., Kumar, S., Jerina, D. M., and Conney, A. H. Biological activity of benzo(e)pyrene. *J. Biol. Chem.*, **254**, 4408–4415 (1979).
34. Wood, A. W., Levin, W., Thomas, P. E., Ryan, D., Karle, J. M., Yagi, H., Jerina, D. M., and Conney, A. H. Metabolic activation of dibenzo(a, h)anthracene and its dihydrodiols to bacterial mutagens. *Cancer Res.*, **38**, 1967–1973 (1978).
35. Watanabe, J., Kawajiri, K., Yonekawa, H., Nagao, M., and Tagashira, Y. Immunological analysis of the roles of two major types of cytochrome P-450 in mutagenesis of compounds isolated from pyrolysates. *Biochem. Biophys. Res. Commun.*, **104**, 193–199 (1982).

ACTIVATION OF CARCINOGENIC COMPOUNDS BY PURIFIED CYTOCHROME P-450 IN RECONSTITUTED SYSTEMS

Tetsuya KAMATAKI and Ryuichi KATO

*Department of Pharmacology, School of Medicine, Keio University**

Enzymatic mechanisms responsible for the mutagenic activation of promutagens including amino acid pyrolysis products were studied using forms of cytochrome P-450 purified from liver microsomes of rats. It was found that 3-amino-1-methyl-5H-pyrido(4, 3-*b*) indole and other promutagens in pyrolysates were rather specifically activated to mutagens by a high-spin form of cytochrome P-450 purified from liver microsomes of polychlorinated biphenyl-treated rats, as compared to other forms purified from phenobarbital and polycholrinated biphenyl-treated rats. The high-spin form of cytochrome P-450 also activated other known promutagens such as 4-aminobiphenyl, 2-aminofluorene, and aflatoxin B_1 at higher rates than did the other forms: cytochrome b_5 was required for its full activities.

This cytochrome was assumed to play central roles in the activation of these promutagens, since this hemoprotein existed as one of the major forms of cytochrome P-450 in liver microsomes of polychlorinated biphenyl-treated rats.

Most carcinogens undergo metabolic transformation to form reactive metabolites, which themselves can bind to DNA or are subject to further process of metabolic activation. Cytochrome P-450 has been recognized to be a group of enzymes catalyzing the formation of the metabolites. Thus, its involvement in the formation of mutagens from benzo[a]pyrene (*21, 30*), 2-acetylaminofluorene (*7*), and other limited promutagens (*21*) has been demonstrated using the reconstituted system containing purified preparations of cytochrome P-450.

Sugimura and his associates have discovered potent promutagens in food pyrolysates (*15, 26–28*). The mutagenicities of some of these promutagens were estimated to be several hundred times as high as benzo[a]pyrene calculated on the basis of μg of the promutagens. The carcinogenicities as well as mutagenicities of these compounds have also been proved. Most of these promutagens exert their mutagenicities after they undergo metabolic transformation by enzymes present in the $9,000 \times g$ supernatant fraction of liver homogenates from polychlorinated biphenyl (PCB)-treated rats. Despite these studies, the exact enzymatic mechanisms responsible for the activation of these promutagens were unknown.

Thus, we initiated this study to clarify the enzymatic mechanisms by which these new promutagens were activated. We report herein that among forms of cytochrome

---

* Shinanomachi 35, Shinjuku-ku, Tokyo 160, Japan (鎌滝哲也, 加藤隆一).

P-450 a high-spin form plays a central role in the mutagen production from several promutagens including those isolated from amino acid and protein pyrolysates.

Involvement of Cytochrome P-450 in the Activation of Promutagens Isolated from Tryptophan Pyrolysate

Potent promutagens, 3-amino-1,4-dimethyl-5H-pyrido(4,3-*b*)indole (Trp-P-1) and 3-amino-1-methyl-5H-pyrido(4,3-*b*)indole (Trp-P-2) were isolated from pyrolysate of tryptophan (*16, 25*). Since liver 9,000×*g* supernatant fraction contains numerous enzymes, we examined the intracellular localization of enzymes responsible for the activation of the promutagens. The results showed that most of the enzymes, if not all, were located in the microsomal but not the cytosolic fraction (*6*). The enzymes required NADPH rather than NADH for their activities and were inhibited by carbon monoxide, suggesting that cytochrome P-450 in liver microsomes was involved in the activation. The microsomal activities were inhibited by α-naphthoflavone and other compounds (*6*), known inhibitors of 3-methylcholanthrene (MC)-inducible forms of cytochrome P-450. In other studies, we clarified that Trp-P-2 was N-hydroxylated at 3-position to exhibit its mutagenicity (*31, 32*) and to bind to DNA (*18*). Also proved was that the N-hydroxylation was the rate limiting step in the possible activation processes in rat hepatocytes (*19*).

There are strains of mice which show different responses to MC in their activities of arylhydrocarbon (benzo[a]pyrene) hydroxylase. The enzyme in C57BL/6N (B6) mice is induced, while that in DBA/2N (D2) mice is not induced, by MC. In our studies, treatment of B6 mice induced the activities of mutagen production and N-hydroxylation of Trp-P-2 as well as the activity of benzo[a]pyrene hydroxylation, whereas the treatment of D2 mice did not induce any of the activities (*34*). Therefore, we tentatively confirmed that an identical form of cytochrome P-450 catalyzed benzo[a]pyrene hydroxylation and Trp-P-2 activation. Forms of cytochrome P-450 which are active in benzo[a]pyrene hydroxylation have been purified from liver microsomes of rats (*2, 17, 23, 24*) and mice (*20*).

Reconstitution of the Activities of Mutagen Production and N-hydroxylation of Trp-P-2 with Purified Cytochrome P-450

A low-spin form of cytochrome P-450 of rats, P-450c purified by Ryan *et al.* (*23*) and P-450$_{\beta NF/ISF-G}$ by Guengerich *et al.* (*2*), is shown to exhibit high benzo[a]pyrene hydroxylation activity. Viewing the results mentioned above, we believed that our preparation of cytochrome P-450, P-448 II-d which is presumably identical to P-450c, was capable of activating Trp-P-2 at a much higher rate than the other forms. We found that P-448 II-d did show higher activities in mutagenic activation and N-hydroxylation of Trp-P-2 than did the other forms of cytochrome P-450 purified from phenobarbital- or PCB-treated rats (*5*).

It has become a general concept that a purified preparation of cytochrome P-450 shows a higher turnover number in oxidizing a drug substrate if the substrate is very specific to the cytochrome. There are two possibilities which may account for this fact. One is that in the reconstituted system we add excess amounts of NADPH-cytochrome

P-450 reductase which could be one of the rate limiting enzymes for drug oxidations in liver microsomes. It has been reported that only about one-tenth of the amount of the reductase exists in liver microsomes as in those of cytochrome P-450 on the molar basis (1). Another possible reason for the increment of specific activity of cytochrome P-450 is that it is caused only by the elimination of forms which are actually inactive for a certain reaction during the purification. Although we found higher activity with P-448 II-d, which was in accordance with our earlier findings, the specific activity of P-448 II-d in the mutagenic activation of Trp-P-2 was only comparable to that of total cytochrome P-450 in liver microsomes of PCB-treated rats (5, 6).

Purification and Characterization of a High-spin Form of Cytochrome P-450 (P-448 II-a) with High Activity in Trp-P-2 Activation

Since the mutagen-producing ability of P-448 II-d was lower than expected, we looked for a form(s) of cytochrome P-450 having higher activity. The purification procedure for four forms of cytochrome P-450 is summarized in Fig. 1. With modifications in the components of the buffers reported by Imai and Sato (4), we divided forms of cytochrome P-450 into two fractions, I and II (11), by ω-amino-n-octyl Sepharose 4B column. The I fraction showed a peak at 450.0 nm while the II fraction showed one at 447.5 nm in the reduced-carbon monoxide binding spectra. Further purification steps with DE-52 and hydroxylapatite columns allowed us to isolate four electrophoretically homogeneous preparations of cytochrome P-450, P-450 I-c, P-450 I-d, P-448 II-a, and P-448 II-d (12). Molecular weights estimated by SDS-polyacrylamide gel electrophoresis were 52,500, 53,000, 54,000, and 56,000, and peaks in the reduced-carbon monoxide binding spectra were at 449.5, 450.5, 447.0, and 447.0 nm for P-450 I-c, P-450 I-d, P-448 II-a, and P-448 II-d, respectively. P-448 II-a showed a peak

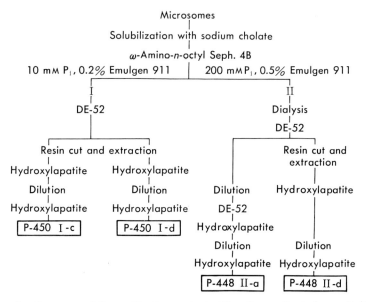

FIG. 1.   Summary of the purification method of four forms of cytochrome P-450 from liver microsomes of PCB-treated rats.

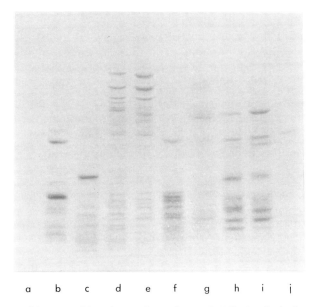

a   b   c   d   e   f   g   h   i   j

Fig. 2.   Peptide maps of four forms of cytochrome P-450 after limited proteolysis
with chymotrypsin. Purified preparations of P-450 I-c (wells e and i), P-450 I-d
(wells d and h), P-448 II-a (wells b and f), and P-448 II-d (wells c and g) were
treated with chymotrypsin (a-e) or papain (f-j) and applied to SDS-polyacrylamide
gel electrophoresis. Chymotrypsin (a) or papain (j) alone was applied as a
control.

at 393 nm while other forms showed it at 416–417 nm in absolute spectra, indicating that
only P-448 II-a is in a high-spin state. Judging from the molecular weights, spectral
properties and other properties, we assume that P-450 I-c, P-450 I-d, P-448 II-a, and
P-448 II-d are identical with the P-450 PB4, P-450 PB5 of Waxman and Walsh (29),
P-450d and P-450c of Ryan et al. (23), respectively. The structural similarities and
dissimilarities among these four forms of cytochrome P-450 were examined by analyzing
peptide maps (Fig. 2). Upon limited proteolysis with chymotrypsin, peptide maps of
P-450 I-c and P-450 I-d showed striking similarities, whereas distinct peptide maps
were obtained among P-450 I-c, P-448 II-a, and P-448 II-d. In agreement with the
analysis of peptide maps, antibodies to P-450 I-c and P-450 I-d cross-reacted with each
other to respectively form fused precipitation lines with P-450 I-d and P-450 I-c in
Ouchterlony double-diffusion analysis. These antibodies, however, did not react with
P-448 II-a and P-448 II-d. Antibodies to P-448 II-a partially cross-reacted with P-448
II-d as previously noted by Reik et al. (22) using P-450c and P-450d.

Spin states of cytochrome P-450 are readily changed with temperature, ionic
strength of media, and binding with a substrate. Thus, it was possible to assume that
the high-spin state of P-448 II-a was caused by PCB which remained bound to this
hemoprotein. To examine this possibility, PCB was extracted from the purified preparation and subjected to gas chromatography. Although not shown here, we found
that only trace amounts of PCB were bound to purified preparations of P-448 II-a
and P-448 II-d. Comparable amounts of peaks were detected in both P-448 preparations, and the amounts were calculated to be less than 1% of the cytochromes on a molar

basis. Therefore, it was confirmed that the high-spin state of P-448 II-a was not caused by the bound PCB.

Catalytic Activities of Purified Forms of Cytochrome P-450

The catalytic activities of the purified preparations of cytochrome P-450 were compared by reconstitution with NADPH-cytochrome P-450 reductase. As can be seen in Table I, each form of cytochrome P-450 showed some substrate specificity. P-450 I-c showed higher activities in aniline p-hydroxylation, and hexobarbital 3-hydroxylation. P-448 II-a catalyzed the O-dealkylations of p-alkoxyaniline derivatives, while P-448 II-d catalyzed the O-dealkylations of p-alkoxynitrobenzene derivatives. It is interesting to note that the p-alkoxy-derivatives with a longer alkyl chain are better substrates for both P-448 II-a and P-448 II-d. P-448 II-d showed higher activities with hydroxylation of biphenyl and benzo[a]pyrene. P-450 I-c also showed high activities with hydroxylation of biphenyl at 4-position and benzo[a]pyrene. Unlike P-448 II-a, P-450 I-c was a poor catalyst for biphenyl 2-hydroxylation.

The mutagen-producing activities of the four forms of cytochrome P-450 were examined (Table II). The P-448 forms catalyzed the mutagenic activation of aflatoxin B$_1$, 2-aminofluorene, and 3-methoxy-4-aminoazobenzene more efficiently than did the

TABLE I. Substrate Specificity of Four Forms of Cytochrome P-450 Purified from Liver Microsomes of PCB-treated Rats

Substrate	Cytochrome P-450			
	I-c	I-d	II-a	II-d
		(nmol/nmol P-450/min)		
Aniline	1.08	0.30	0.85	0.33
p-Methoxyaniline	0.38	0.38	0.85	0.55
p-Ethoxyaniline	0.39	0.50	3.30	1.37
p-Propoxyaniline	0.64	1.33	3.53	1.35
p-Methoxynitrobenzene	0.69	0.08	0.17	1.15
p-Ethoxynitrobenzene	1.47	1.41	3.28	12.39
p-Propoxynitrobenzene	2.72	1.82	6.87	34.97
Biphenyl (2-OH)	0.25	0.22	2.21	2.93
(4-OH)	3.40	0.83	2.52	3.77
Hexobarbital 3-OH	1.80	0.51	0.03	0.15
Benzo[a]pyrene	2.59	0.88	0.07	4.33

TABLE II. Mutagenic Activation of Promutagens by Purified Preparations of Cytochrome P-450 from Liver Microsomes of PCB-treated Rats

Promutagen	S. typhimurium	Cytochrome P-450			
		I-c	I-d	II-a	II-d
			(Rev./plate)		
Aflatoxin B$_1$	TA100	29	109	817	173
Benzo[a]pyrene	TA100	38	135	84	222
2-Aminofluorene	TA98	65	77	1,266	567
3-Methoxy-4-aminoazobenzene	TA98	38	109	324	268

P-450 forms. P-450 I-d showed a higher activity in the activation of benzo[a]pyrene than did P-450 I-c. As stated, P-450 I-c was a better catalyst than P-450 I-d for hydroxylations of benzo[a]pyrene. Thus, P-450 I-c and P-450 I-d catalyze the oxidation of benzo[a]pyrene at different positions. P-448 II-a and P-448 II-d showed higher rates of activation of other mutagens as depicted below.

Comparison of P-448 Forms in the Capacities of Mutagenic Activation

Considerable interest has been focused on a low-spin form of cytochrome P-450 (P-450c *etc.*, presumably identical to P-448 II-d in this study) because of its high activation of polycyclic hydrocarbons including benzo[a]pyrene. However, we found that P-448 II-a, a distinct form that is identical to P-450d (*10*), is capable of N-hydroxylating Trp-P-2 at a faster rate than P-448 II-d. Thus, P-448 II-a and P-448 II-d were compared to evaluate their toxicological significance with a wide variety of promutagens.

As shown in Table III, Trp-P-2 and Glu-P-1 were N-hydroxylated by P-448 II-a more efficiently than by P-448 II-d. The ratios of the activities of P-448 II-a to those of P-448 II-d for the hydroxylations of Trp-P-2 and Glu-P-1 were about 3 and 45, respectively, indicating that Glu-P-1 rather than Trp-P-2 was a specific substrate for the high-spin cytochrome. P-448 II-a was also a better catalyst for the N-hydroxylations of 2-aminofluorene and 4-aminobiphenyl. Acetanilide, a known substrate for a high-spin form of cytochrome P-450 isolated from rabbit livers, was hydroxylated by P-448 II-a at about 1.6-fold higher rate than by P-448 II-d.

The N-hydroxylation of Trp-P-2 and Glu-P-1 is recognized to be a common activation process to exert their mutagenicities. In agreement with this concept, these promutagens were activated to mutagens by the high-spin form more efficiently than

TABLE III.   Comparison of the Activities of P-448 II-a and P-448 II-d to
Hydroxylate Foreign Compounds Including Promutagens

Substrate	Reaction	P-448		P-448 II-a/ P-448 II-d
		II-a	II-d	
		(nmol/nmol P-448/min)		
Trp-P-1	N-OH	2.09	0.70	2.99
Glu-P-1	N-OH	3.93	0.09	44.7
2-Aminofluorene	N-OH	16.30	2.14	7.62
4-Aminobiphenyl	N-OH	38.10	1.70	22.4
Acetanilide	4-OH	14.91	9.28	1.61

TABLE IV.   Comparison of P-448 II-a and P-448 II-d in the Mutagenic
Activation of Promutagens

Promutagen	*S. typhimurium*	P-448 II-a	P-448 II-d
		(Rev. $\times 10^3$/nmol P-448)	
Trp-P-2	TA98	7,810	3,650
Glu-P-1	TA98	5,090	180
IQ	TA98	2,410	202
2-Acetylaminofluorene	TA98	5.05	1.43
4-Aminobiphenyl	TA98	11.50	1.58

by the low-spin form (Table IV). It was also shown that Glu-P-1 was activated specifically by the high-spin cytochrome. In addition, 2-amino-3-methylimidazo[4,5-*f*]quinoline (IQ), which was isolated from pyrolysates of charred parts of sardine and beefsteak (*13*, *14*), was activated by P-448 II-a rather specifically (*33*). 2-Acetylaminofluorene is known to be activated to a mutagen(s) by a high-spin form of cytochrome P-450 purified from rabbit liver. This promutagen induced higher numbers of revertants after undergoing metabolic transformation by P-448 II-a.

Characteristic Requirement of Cytochrome b_5 for Maximum Activities of P-448 II-a

During the examination of the catalytic activities of P-448 II-a, we found that this enzyme required cytochrome b_5 for its maximum activities. Table V shows the effects of added cytochrome b_5 on oxidations of a variety of substrates. Cytochrome b_5 enhanced the activity of P-448 II-a in all reactions examined except in coumarin 7-hydroxylation in which no significant activity was observed. The magnitude of the enhancement was apparently dependent on the structure of substrates. The length of alkyl chain to be oxidized and other portions such as amino and nitro groups affected the enhancement as well as the O-dealkylation activity. In contrast to P-448 II-a, no, or only trace, amounts of enhancement were seen when P-448 II-d was used.

The mechanisms by which cytochrome b_5 enhanced the activity of P-448 II-a were studied with *p*-propoxyaniline as a substrate (*9*). The maximum enhancement was attainable when the ratio of cytochrome b_5 to P-448 II-a was 0.5 on a molar basis. Hildebrandt and Estabrook (*3*) demonstrated that cytochrome b_5 can transport the second of two electrons to cytochrome P-450 to oxidize a drug. Thereafter, we demonstrated the possibility that cytochrome b_5 could transfer two electrons required for drug oxidation catalyzed by cytochrome P-450 (*8*). Thus, cytochrome b_5 was assumed to act as an electron carrier to P-448 II-a. In accordance with this idea, when smaller amounts of NADPH-cytochrome P-450 reductase were added to the reconstituted system, greater enhancement was observed. Despite this observation, 100% enhance-

TABLE V. Effects of Cytochrome b_5 on the Activities of P-448 II-a and P-448 II-d

Substrate	P-448 II-a	P-448 II-d
	(% enhancement)	
Aniline	+213	+ 9
p-Methoxyaniline	+ 52	+ 5
p-Ethoxyaniline	+ 46	− 5
p-Propoxyaniline	+103	−10
p-Methoxynitrobenzene	+ 53	+35
p-Ethoxynitrobenzene	+156	+26
p-Propoxynitrobenzene	+227	+15
Coumarin	0	0
7-Methoxycoumarin	+309	0
7-Ethoxycoumarin	+162	+ 5
7-Propoxycoumarin	+102	+10
7-Isopropoxycoumarin	+266	+ 4
7-Buthoxycoumarin	+ 94	+ 2

ment remained even when excess amounts of the reductase were added. These results probably indicate that two mechanisms are involved in the facilitation of electron transfer by cytochrome b_5 from NADPH to P-448 II-a. The possibility of whether cytochrome b_5 changes the affinity of P-448 II-a to bind with a substrate was examined with various concentrations of p-propoxyaniline. Results showed that the addition of cytochrome b_5 increased the affinity of P-448 II-a to the substrate. Cytochrome b_5 decreased the K_m value to about a half and approximately doubled V_{max} value. These results suggest that cytochrome b_5 enhances the activity of P-448 II-a by multiple mechanisms. These mechanisms may be the cause of the enhancement variations noted with the forms of cytochrome P-450 and substrates employed.

Enhancement by cytochrome b_5 of the activities of P-448 II-a may affect the ability of this hemoprotein to activate promutagens. In fact, the addition of cytochrome b_5 enhanced the production of mutagens (10). As shown in Table VI, the mutagen-producing activities of P-448 II-a from Glu-P-1, 2-aminofluorene, and 3-methoxy-4-aminoazobenzene were increased by about 56, 65, and 87%, respectively.

As mentioned above, the specific activity of P-448 II-a in the mutagenic activation of several promutagens was the highest among four forms of cytochrome P-450 purified from PCB-treated rats. Thus, another thing was to quantify the amounts of this form of cytochrome P-450 in liver microsomes to evaluate its toxicological significance. Using monospecific antibodies to P-448 II-a, we quantified the amounts by the radial immunodiffusion method (10). As shown in Fig. 3, only a trace amount of P-448 II-a was detected in liver microsomes of untreated male rats, while it existed in larger amounts in liver microsomes of female rats. Treatment of male rats with PCB dramatically increased the amount, which accounted for about 50% of total cytochrome

TABLE VI. Enhancement by Cytochrome b_5 of the Mutagen-producing Activities of P-448 II-a

Promutagen	Concn. (mM)	$-b_5$	$+b_5$	Change (%)
		(Rev. $\times 10^{-3}$/nmol P-448 II-a)		
Glu-P-1	0.02	126	197	$+56$
2-Aminofluorene	0.2	12.7	21.0	$+65$
3-Methoxy-4-aminoazobenzene	0.2	3.74	6.07	$+87$

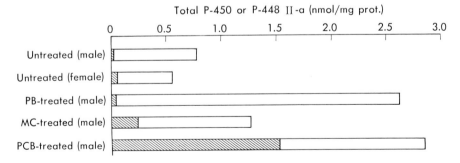

FIG. 3. Radial immunodiffusion assay of rat liver microsomes for the content of P-448 II-a using purified anti-P-448 II-a IgG-impregnated agarose gels.

P-450 in liver microsomes. MC also increased P-448 II-a but the extent of induction was less than that seen with PCB.

In conclusion, we found that P-448 II-a rather than P-448 II-d showed higher activities in transforming some promutagens including Trp-P-2 and Glu-P-1 to mutagens. The activities of P-448 II-a were enhanced by cytochrome b_5. The toxicological significance of P-448 II-a was confirmed by the fact that it existed in larger amounts in liver microsomes of PCB- or MC-treated rats.

REFERENCES

1. Estabrook, R. W. and Werringloer, J. Chairman's introductory statement: The microsomal system responsible for the oxidative metabolism of many drugs. *In* "The Induction of Drug Metabolism," ed. R. W. Estabrook and E. Lindenlaub, pp. 187–199 (1978). F. K. Schattauer Verlag, Stuttgart and New York.

2. Guengerich, F. P., Dannan, G. A., Wright, S. T., Martin, M. V., and Kaminsky, L. S. Purification and characterization of liver microsomal cytochromes P-450: Electrophoretic, spectral, catalytic, and immunochemical properties and inducibility of eight isozymes isolated from rats treated with phenobarbital and β-naphthoflavone. *Biochemistry*, **21**, 6019–6030 (1982).

3. Hildebrandt, A. and Estabrook, R. W. Evidence for the participation of cytochrome b_5 in hepatic microsomal mixed-function oxidation reactions. *Arch. Biochem. Biophys.*, **143**, 66–79 (1971).

4. Imai, Y. and Sato, R. An affinity column method for partial purification of cytochrome P-450 from phenobarbital-induced rabbit liver microsomes. *J. Biochem.*, **75**, 689–697 (1974).

5. Ishii, K., Ando, M., Kamataki, T., and Kato, R. Metabolic activation of mutagenic tryptophan pyrolysis products (Trp-P-1 and Trp-P-2) by a purified cytochrome P-450-dependent monooxygenase system. *Cancer Lett.*, **9**, 271–276 (1980).

6. Ishii, K., Yamazoe, Y., Kamataki, T., and Kato, R. Metabolic activation of mutagenic tryptophan pyrolysis products by rat liver microsomes. *Cancer Res.*, **40**, 2596–2600 (1980).

7. Johnson, E. F., Levitt, D. S., Muller-Eberhard, U., and Thorgeirsson, S. S. Catalysis of divergent pathways of 2-acetylaminofluorene metabolism by multiple forms of cytochrome P-450. *Cancer Res.*, **40**, 4456–4459 (1980).

8. Kamataki, T. and Kitagawa, H. The involvement of cytochrome P-450 in the NADH-dependent O-demethylation of p-nitroanisole in phenobarbital-treated rabbit liver microsomes. *Biochem. Biophys. Res. Commun.*, **76**, 1007–1013 (1977).

9. Kamataki, T., Maeda, K., Matsuda, N., Ishii, K., Yamazoe, Y., and Kato, R. A high spin form of cytochrome P-448 highly purified from PCB-treated rats. II. Characteristic requirement of cytochrome b_5 for maximum activity. *Biochem. Pharmacol.*, **32**, 2479–2483 (1983).

10. Kamataki, T., Maeda, K., Yamazoe, Y., Matsuda, N., Ishii, K., and Kato, R. A high spin form of cytochrome P-450 highly purified from PCB-treated rats: Catalytic characterization and immunochemical quantitation in liver microsomes. *Mol. Pharmacol.*, **24**, 146–155 (1983).

11. Kamataki, T., Maeda, K., Yamazoe, Y., Nagai, T., and Kato, R. Partial purification and characterization of cytochrome P-450 responsible for the occurrence of sex difference in drug metabolism in the rat. *Biochem. Biophys. Res. Commun.*, **103**, 1–7 (1981).

12. Kamataki, T., Yoshizawa, H., Ishii, K., and Kato, R. Separation and purification of

multiple forms of cytochrome P-450 from PCB-treated rats and human livers. *In* "Microsomes, Drug Oxidations and Drug Toxicity," ed. R. Sato and R. Kato, pp. 99–100 (1982). Japan Sci. Soc. Press, Tokyo / Wiley-Interscience, New York.

13. Kasai, H., Nishimura, S., Wakabayashi, K., Nagao, M., and Sugimura, T. Chemical synthesis of 2-amino-3-methyl-imidazo[4, 5-*f*]quinoline (IQ), a potent mutagen isolated from broiled fish. *Proc. Jpn. Acad.*, **56B**, 382–384 (1980).

14. Kasai, H., Yamaizumi, Z., Nishimura, S., Wakabayashi, K., Nagao, M., Sugimura, T., Yokoyama, S., and Miyazawa, T. A potent mutagen in broiled fish. Part 1. 2-Amino-3-methyl-3*H*-imidazo[4, 5*f*]quinoline. *J. Chem. Soc., Parkin*, **1**, 2290–2293 (1981).

15. Kawachi, T., Nagao, M., Yahagi, T., Takahashi, Y., Sugimura, T., Takayama, S., Kosuge, T., and Shudo, T. Mutagens and carcinogens in food. *In* "Advances in Medical Oncology, Research and Education," ed. G. P. Margison, Vol. 1, pp. 199–206 (1979). Pergamon Press, New York.

16. Kosuge, T., Tsuji, K., Wakabayashi, K., Okamoto, T., Shudo, K., Iitaka, Y., Itai, A., Sugimura, T., Kawachi, T., Nagao, M., Yahagi, T., and Seino, Y. Isolation and structure studies of mutagenic principles in amino acid pyrolysates. *Chem. Pharm. Bull.*, **26**, 611–619 (1978).

17. Lau, P. P. and Strobel, H. W. Multiple forms of cytochrome P-450 in liver microsomes from β-naphthoflavone-pretreated rats. Separation, purification, and characterization of five forms. *J. Biol. Chem.*, **257**, 5257–5262 (1982).

18. Mita, S., Ishii, K., Yamazoe, Y., Kamataki, T., Kato, R., and Sugimura, T. Evidence for the involvement of N-hydroxylation of 3-amino-1-methyl-5*H*-pyrido[4,3*b*]indole by cytochrome P-450 in the covalent binding to DNA. *Cancer Res.*, **41**, 3610–3614 (1981).

19. Mita, S., Yamazoe, Y., Kamataki, T., and Kato, R. Metabolic activation of Trp-P-2, a tryptophan-pyrolysis mutagen, by isolated rat hepatocytes. *Biochem. Pharmacol.*, **32**, 1179–1182 (1983).

20. Negishi, M. and Nebert, D. W. Structural gene product of the *Ah* locus. Genetic and immunochemical evidence for two forms of mouse liver cytochrome P-450 induced by 3-methylcholanthrene. *J. Biol. Chem.*, **254**, 11015–11023 (1979).

21. Norman, R. L., Muller-Eberhard, U., and Johnson, E. F. The role of cytochrome P-450 forms in 2-aminoanthracene and benzo(a)pyrene mutagenesis. *Biochem. Biophys. Res. Commun.*, **89**, 195–201 (1979).

22. Reik, L. M., Levin, W., Ryan, D. E., and Thomas, P. E. Immunochemical relatedness of rat hepatic microsomal cytochrome P-450c and P-450d. *J. Biol. Chem.*, **257**, 3950–3957 (1982).

23. Ryan, D. E., Thomas, P. E., Korzeniowski, D., and Levin, W. Separation and characterization of highly purified forms of liver microsomal cytochrome P-450 from rats treated with polychlorinated biphenyls, phenobarbital and 3-methylcholanthrene. *J. Biol. Chem.*, **254**, 1365–1374 (1979).

24. Saito, T. and Strobel, H. W. Purification to homogeneity and characterization of a form of cytochrome P-450 with high specificity for benzo(a)pyrene from β-naphthoflavone-pretreated rat liver microsomes. *J. Biol. Chem.*, **256**, 984–988 (1981).

25. Sugimura, T., Kawachi, T., Nagao, M., Yahagi, T., Seino, Y., Okamoto, T., Shudo, K., Kosuge, T., Tsuji, K., Wakabayashi, K., Iitaka, T., and Itai, A. Mutagenic principle(s) in tryptophan and phenylalanine pyrolysis products. *Proc. Jpn. Acad.*, **53**, 58–61 (1977).

26. Sugimura, T., Nagao, M., Kawachi, T., Honda, M., Yahagi, T., Seino, Y., Sato, S., Matsukura, N., Matsushima, T., Shirai, A., Sawamura, M., and Matsumoto, H. Mutagen-carcinogens in food with special reference to highly mutagenic pyrolytic products in broiled foods. *In* "Origins of Human Cancer," ed. H. H. Hiatt, J. D. Watson, and

J. A. Winsten, pp. 1561–1577 (1977). Cold Spring Harbor Laboratory, New York.

27. Sugimura, T. and Nagao, M. Mutagenic factors in cooked food. *CRC Crit. Rev. Toxicol.*, **6**, 189–209 (1979).

28. Sugimura, T., Wakabayashi, K., Yamada, M., Nagao, M., and Fujino, T. Activation of chemicals to proximal carcinogens. *In* "Mechanisms of Toxicity and Hazard Evaluation," ed. B. Holmstedt, R. Lauwerys, M. Mercier, and M. Roberfroid, pp. 205–217 (1980). Elsevier/North-Holland Biomedical Press, Amsterdam.

29. Waxman, D. J. and Walsh, C. Phenobarbital-induced rat liver cytochrome P-450. Purification and characterization of two closely related isozymic forms. *J. Biol. Chem.*, **257**, 10446–10457 (1982).

30. Wood, A. W., Levin, W., Lu, A.Y.H., Yagi, H., Hernandez, O., Jerina, D. M., and Conney, A. H. Metabolism of benzo(a)pyrene and benzo(a)pyrene derivatives to mutagenic products by highly purified hepatic microsomal enzymes. *J. Biol. Chem.*, **251**, 4882–4890 (1976).

31. Yamazoe, Y., Ishii, K., Kamataki, T., and Kato, R. Isolation and characterization of active metabolites of tryptophan-pyrolysate mutagen, Trp-P-2, formed by rat liver microsomes. *Chem.-Biol. Interact.*, **30**, 125–138 (1980).

32. Yamazoe, Y., Ishii, K., Kamataki, T., and Kato, R. Structural elucidation of a mutagenic metabolite of 3-amino-1-methyl-5*H*-pyrido[4,3*b*]indole. *Drug Metab. Dispos.*, **9**, 292–296 (1981).

33. Yamazoe, Y., Shimada, M., Kamataki, T., and Kato, R. Microsomal activation of 2-amino-3-methylimidazo[4,5*f*]quinoline, a pyrolysate of sardine and beef extracts, to a mutagenic intermediate. *Cancer Res.*, **43**, 5768–5774 (1983).

34. Yamazoe, Y., Yamaguchi, N., Kamataki, T., and Kato, R. Metabolic activation of Trp-P-2, a mutagenic amine from tryptophan-pyrolysate, by liver microsomes from 3-methylcholanthrene-responsive and non-responsive mice. *Xenobiotica*, **10**, 483–494 (1980).

GANN Monograph on Cancer Research 30, 1985

MECHANISM OF METABOLIC ACTIVATION OF CARCINOGENIC AROMATIC AMINES

Chikayoshi NAGATA, Masahiko KODAMA, Teruyuki KIMURA, and Tsutomu NAKAYAMA

*Biophysics Division, National Cancer Center Research Institute**

Evidence has been presented implicating the causal significance of free radicals in the carcinogenesis of aromatic amines. Thus, enzymatically formed proximate carcinogens of aminoazo dyes and naphthylamines were found to be easily converted into the corresponding free radicals. When aminoazo dyes were incubated with liver microsomes from rats treated with 3-methylcholanthrene (MC-microsomes), nitroxide radicals produced from the dyes were detected, and an intimate correlation was found between the free radical formation and the hepatocarcinogenicity of the aminoazo dyes, indicating that the N-hydroxylation was the rate-determining step of carcinogenesis.

When 2-naphthylamine (2-NA) was incubated with MC-microsomes, an ESR signal was observed. It was identified as a mixture of free radicals produced from N-hydroxy-2-naphthylamine (N-OH-2-NA) and 2-amino-1-naphthol. An ESR signal of the same magnitude as that with MC-microsomes was observed with liver microsomes from rats treated with phenobarbital (PB-microsomes), but the signal pattern was different from that with MC-microsomes. This difference was a reflection of the different metabolic pathways of 2-NA in the two microsomes. With untreated microsomes the ESR signal was much smaller. The free radicals produced from aminoazo dyes and 2-NA were sufficiently reactive to bind covalently to DNA.

The cytochrome P-450 enzyme systems were found to catalyze both the N-hydroxylation and ring-hydroxylation of aminoazo dyes and naphthylamines, while the flavine-containing monooxygenase catalyzed only the N-hydroxylation. MC-induced P-448 was exclusively involved in generating the nitroxide radical from the aminoazo dyes in the cytochrome P-450 system, whereas both MC-induced P-448 and PB-induced P-450 were involved in generating the free radicals from naphthylamines. Accompanying the free radical formation, active oxygens such as hydrogen peroxide and superoxide anion radical were generated, implying the causal significance of concomitant formation of free radical and active oxygen in the carcinogenesis of aromatic amines.

The success of Yamagiwa and Ichikawa in producing tumors in rabbits by applying coal tar (*48*), prompted the isolation of the carcinogenic compounds from that source. Benzo[a]pyrene was identified as the principal carcinogenic factor involved (*4*).

---

* Tsukiji 5-1-1, Chuo-ku, Tokyo 104, Japan (永田親義, 児玉昌彦, 木村晃之, 中山　勉).

Since then extensive work has been carried out to detect and isolate carcinogenic substances, and many kinds of chemical carcinogens such as polycyclic aromatic hydrocarbons, aromatic amines, alkylating agents, *etc.* have been found. In this sense, the former half of this century can be said to be "an age of discovery of chemical carcinogens." Since 1960, the main concern of researchers in this field has been the molecular mechanism of tumor production by chemical carcinogens. The discovery of cytochrome P-450 has initiated a new aspect in chemical carcinogenesis.

In this article, the carcinogenic mechanism of aromatic amines such as aminoazo dyes and naphthylamines is treated. The aminoazo dyes and the aromatic hydrocarbons have been most studied (*1, 29*). However, details of the mechanism of tumor production remain unsolved. Naphthylamines have attracted much attention because of their carcinogenicity in man. Although occupational bladder cancer caused by 2-naphthylamine (2-NA) has progressively decreased due to the severe restriction of industrial use, human exposure to this carcinogen still continues because it was detected in cigarette smoke (*37*) and the increased risk of bladder cancer in smokers was partly ascribed to it (*47*). Previously it was discovered that benzo[a]pyrene was activated by the cytochrome P-450 system to form 6-hydroxybenzo[a]pyrene and that this metabolite was easily converted to the 6-oxybenzo[a]pyrene radical (*30, 32, 34*). This radical was found to be further oxidized to benzo[a]pyrene-quinones. Since the benzo[a]pyrene-semiquinone radical was sufficiently reactive to bind to DNA (*24, 31*), the pathway of 6-oxybenzo[a]pyrene radical formation was thought to be one of the activation pathways of benzo[a]pyrene (*32, 34, 44*). Similarly, aminoazo dyes and naphthylamines have been found to be metabolized by the cytochrome P-450 system and/or flavine-containing monooxygenase (FMO) to proximate forms which were easily converted to free radicals. These free radicals were sufficiently reactive to bind to DNA. In view of these findings, the free radical reaction mechanism in carcinogenesis of aromatic amines is proposed.

Aminoazo Dyes

1. *Free radical formation from aminoazo dyes*

The mode of tumor production by aminoazo dyes differs from that of polycyclic aromatic hydrocarbons in that the former produce tumors at a point remote from the site of application. This suggests that metabolism is crucial in eliciting tumors and extensive studies on the metabolism of aminoazo dyes have been carried out (*1, 29*). As a result, the major steps in the activation are now well elucidated. Thus, the first step in the activation of N,N-dimethyl-4-aminoazobenzene (DAB) is an oxidative N-demethylation, resulting in the formation of N-methyl-4-aminoazobenzene (MAB) (*29*). This reaction is catalyzed by both cytochrome P-450 and FMO (*8, 46, 49*). The second step is N-hydroxylation to form N-OH-MAB, and this step is considered to be catalyzed by FMO (*14*). N-OH-MAB was considered further metabolized to N-sulfate by sulfotransferase (*15*). Such a pathway of activation was proposed following experiments using liver microsomes from untreated rats (untreated microsomes). However, the metabolic pattern using the liver microsomes from 3-methylcholanthrene-treated rats (MC-microsomes) was different from the pattern with untreated microsomes. Thus, with MC-microsomes, both the P-450 and the FMO systems are involved in the N-hydroxylation of MAB in contrast to the untreated microsomes where FMO alone participates (*14*).

By incubating DAB or MAB with rat liver microsomes at 37° for 10 min, the free radicals were produced, the electron spin resonance (ESR) signals of which are depicted in Fig. 1 a, b (*20*). These signals are all the same indicating that the same free radical species is formed from both DAB and MAB, although the amount from the latter was far greater than that from DAB. Without addition of NADPH to the reaction mixture no ESR signal appeared. NADPH was more effective than NADH in eliciting the ESR signal, and synergistic effects were observed for these two coenzymes.

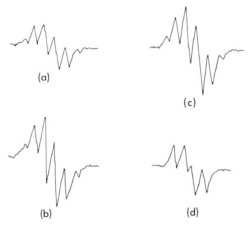

FIG. 1. The ESR signals of the extract of the incubating mixture (37°, 10 min) of aminoazo dyes with MC-microsomes. (a) 3'-methyl-DAB, (b) 3'-methyl-MAB, (c) and (d) are the signals for authentic samples of N-OH-MAB and N-OH-AB, respectively.

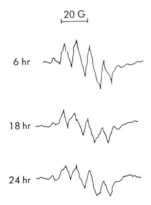

FIG. 2. The ESR signal of the free radical produced from 3'-methyl-DAB *in vivo*. 3'-Methyl-DAB (40 mg/2 ml olive oil) was administered through a stomach tube to male Sprague-Dawley rats (5 weeks old and MC-induced) and after intervals (6, 18, 24 hr), five rats were killed and their livers were homogenized with 8 vol. 0.15 M KCl-0.05 M Tris-HCl buffer (pH 7.5) in polytron for 1 min. After extraction with an equal volume of benzene, the extract was evaporated to dryness and dissolved in 0.3 ml of benzene for the ESR measurement.

When heat-treated (60°, 10 min) microsomes were used, no ESR signal was observed. Carbon monoxide inhibited by 40% the formation of the free radical from 3′-methyl-DAB (CO: air=1: 1) and 80% (CO: air=19: 1). No inhibition was observed for 3′-methyl-MAB (*33*). These results clearly show that the free radicals in Fig. 1, a and b, are produced by the NADPH-dependent cytochrome P-450 system. The same ESR signal was also observed *in vivo* (Fig. 2) (*33*). As the most probable structure of the free radical, the nitroxide radical produced from either N-OH-MAB or N-hydroxy-4-aminoazobenzene (N-OH-AB), which are active metabolites of aminoazo dyes, was supposed. This was tested by ESR measurement after dissolving authentic samples of these metabolites in benzene. The ESR signal of dissolved N-OH-MAB (Fig. 1c) was the same as the signal obtained by incubating DAB or MAB with microsomes (Fig. 1, a, b), indicating that the enzymatically-formed free radical is the nitroxide radical produced from N-OH-MAB (*33*). This identification was further confirmed by simulating the ESR signal with the hyperfine coupling constants calculated by INDO MO (intermediate neglect of differential overlap molecular orbital) method (*33*). It should be stressed that the signal of this nitroxide radical clearly differed from that of the nitroxide radical produced from N-OH-AB which is not considered to be an active metabolite leading to the ultimate carcinogen (*33*). Thus, the scheme of the nitroxide radical formation is proposed as in Fig. 3. As shown in Figs. 4 and 5, good parallelism was observed between the carcinogenicities and the amounts of nitroxide radical formed among a series of DAB and MAB derivatives (*21*). This suggests that the N-hydroxylation of the MAB derivatives leading to the free radical formation is intimately involved in the tumor production by these azo compounds. This suggesting was further supported by the finding that the nitroxide radical covalently binds to DNA (Fig. 6) (*33*). Binding was found to be especially strong with poly G, indicating that the guanine moiety is the binding site. The amount of bound radical of N-OH-AB was far less

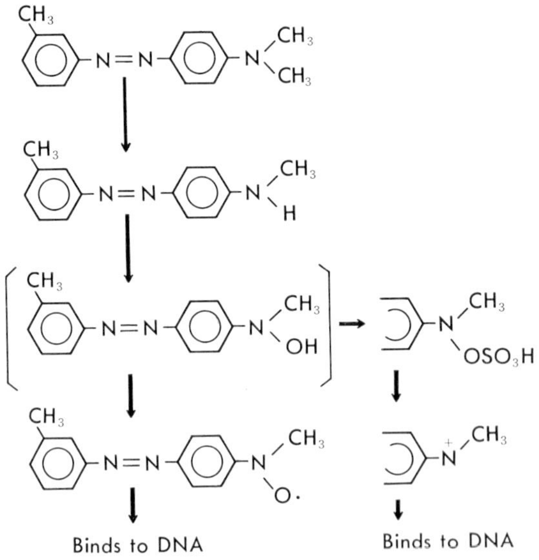

Fig. 3. Proposed metabolic pathways of 3′-methyl-DAB leading to the nitroxide radical.

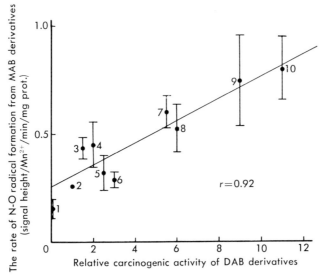

FIG. 4. Correlation between the rate of formation of N-OH-MAB derivatives from DAB derivatives and their hepatocarcinogenicity. Relative carcinogenicity of DAB derivatives is based on the data of Miller and Miller (29). 1, 4'-NO$_2$-DAB; 2, 4'-methyl(Me)-DAB; 3, 4'-Cl-DAB; 4, 2'-Cl-DAB; 5, 2'-Me-DAB; 6, 2'-NO$_2$-DAB; 7, 3'-Cl-DAB; 8, DAB; 9, 3'-NO$_2$-DAB; 10, 3'-Me-DAB.

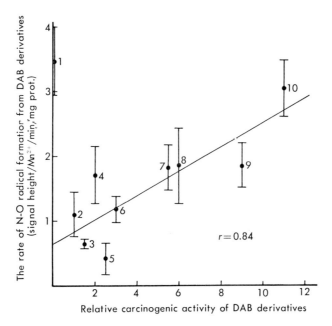

FIG. 5. Correlation between the rate of formation of N-OH-MAB derivatives from MAB derivatives and hepatocarcinogenicity of the corresponding DAB derivatives. 1, 4'-NO$_2$-MAB; 2, 4'-methyl(Me)-MAB; 3, 4'-Cl-MAB; 4, 2'-Cl-MAB; 5, 2'-Me-MAB; 6, 2'-NO$_2$-MAB; 7, 3'-Cl-MAB; 8, MAB; 9, 3'-NO$_2$-MAB; 10, 3'-Me-MAB.

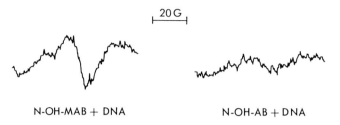

FIG. 6.   ESR signals of the covalently bound adducts of N-OH-MAB or N-OH-
AB with DNA.

than that of N-OH-MAB. Bearing these facts in mind, the free radical formation is
considered to be involved in hepatocarcinogenesis, in addition to the ionic reaction
mechanism presented by Miller (28).

2. Enzyme involved in the metabolism of aminoazo dyes

It has been well established that both cytochrome P-450 and FMO are involved
in the demethylation of DAB to MAB (8, 46, 49). However, no clear conclusion has
been reached concerning the enzymes involved in the metabolic pathways of MAB
to further oxidation products. Kadlubar et al. found that the microsomal N-hydroxylation of MAB was inhibited by 2-[(2,4-dichloro-6-phenyl)phenoxyl]-ethylamine or by
carbon monoxide, and they also observed that the reaction did not occur when cumene
hydroperoxide was used in place of reduced pyridine nucleotide and oxygen (14). From
this, together with the fact that N-OH-MAB was detected when MAB reacted with
purified FMO from porcine liver microsomes, they concluded that the N-hydroxylation
of MAB was independent of cytochrome P-450 and was catalyzed exclusively by FMO
(14). This is considered to be true for untreated microsomes; however, it is not the
case for MC-microsomes. That is, from the viewpoint of free radical formation, the
amount of nitroxide radical with MC-microsomes is extremely large compared with
that with the liver microsomes from phenobarbital-treated rats (PB-microsomes) and
untreated microsomes (Table I). Reflecting this difference in the induction of metabolic
enzymes, the behavior of the enzymes toward various kinds of inhibitors was quite
different from the untreated microsomes. Thus, 1) free radical formation by incubating
MAB with MC-microsomes was not inhibited by such P-450 inhibitors as metyrapone
and SKF-525A, but α-naphthoflavone, which is a specific inhibitor of cytochrome
P-448, considerably inhibited the formation of the nitroxide radical (Fig. 7) (22). 2) The
inhibitory effect of 1-(1-naphthyl)-2-thiourea, an inhibitor of FMO, was quite different depending upon whether the reaction system was partially purified FMO or

TABLE I.   Amounts of Free Radical Formed by Incubating 3'-Methyl-DAB or 3'-Methyl-MAB
with Liver Microsomes from Non-treated, PB-treated, and MC-treated Rats[a]

Substrate	Microsomes		
	Non-treated	PB-treated	MC-treated
3'-Methyl-DAB	0.05 ± 0.01	0.13 ± 0.03	0.59 ± 0.03
3'-Methyl-MAB	0.71 ± 0.03	0.46 ± 0.02	3.10 ± 0.22

[a] The amount of free radical is given by the signal height/Mn^{2+}/mg protein.

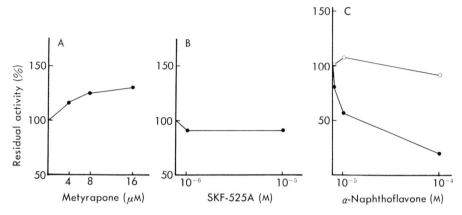

Fig. 7. Effects of metyrapone, SKF-525A, and α-naphthoflavone on the formation of nitroxide radicals from 3′-methyl-MAB.

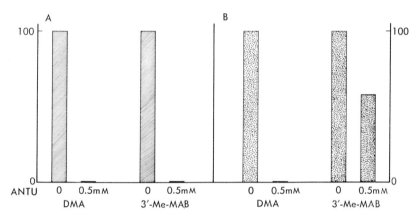

Fig. 8. Effect of 1-(1-naphthyl)-2-thiourea (ANTU) on the N-hydroxylation of 3′-methyl (Me)-MAB and N-oxidation of dimethylaniline (DMA). The amounts of nitroxide radical and dimethylaniline N-oxide without ANTU are taken as 100. A: partially purified FMO. B: microsomes.

microsomes (Fig. 8) (22). Thus, in partially purified FMO, N-hydroxylation of 3′-methyl-MAB as well as N-oxidation of dimethylaniline was inhibited completely by 1-(1-naphthyl)-2-thiourea, whereas the inhibition of N-hydroxylation of 3′-methyl-MAB was only about 40% in the microsomal system. From these results, it appears that, in addition to FMO, the cytochrome P-448 system is involved in the N-hydroxylation of MAB. If this is so, the limited inhibition by carbon monoxide of the N-hydroxylation of 3′-methyl-MAB is difficult to explain. However, this is not inconsistent if we consider the fact that the cytochrome P-448 involved in the N-hydroxylation of aromatic amines is less sensitive to carbon monoxide (27, 43).

The result of the comparative study of metabolism with microsomes and purified enzymes is depicted in Fig. 9. With the reconstituted system of the cytochrome P-450 purified from PB-microsomes (PB-P-450) and cytochrome P-450 reductase, only AB was isolated by high pressure liquid chromatography (HPLC), whereas with FMO from rat liver microsomes (23) only N-OH-MAB was produced (Fig. 9). On the other

C. NAGATA ET AL.

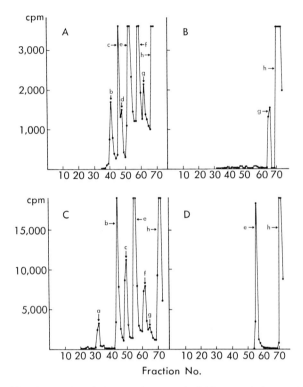

FIG. 9. HPLC profiles of the metabolites of [^{14}C]-MAB (A) with MC-microsomes, (B) with purified MFO, (C) with MC-P-448, and (D) with PB-P-450. a,
4′-OH-AB; b, 3-OH-AB; c, 4′-OH-MAB; d, N-OH-AB; e, AB; f, unknown;
g, N-OH-MAB; h, MAB.

hand, with the reconstituted enzyme system of the cytochrome P-448 purified from
MC-microsomes (MC-P-448) and NADPH-cytochrome P-450 reductase, all metabolites produced with MC-microsomes were detected, although their relative ratios
were not always the same. From these results of HPLC, together with the feature in
the nitroxide radical formation, the enzymes involved in the metabolism of MAB with
MC-microsomes are considered to be as depicted in Fig. 10. Note that both the FMO
and P-450 enzyme systems participate in the production of N-OH-MAB, whereas only
the cytochrome P-450 system is involved in the production of N-OH-AB. Since MAB
is a potent hepatocarcinogen and AB is far less carcinogenic, metabolism leading to
N-OH-MAB has been considered to be the activation pathway in carcinogenesis of
MAB (14, 15). However, this is not true for the activation in mutagenesis. Thus, in the
mutagenesis test, N-OH-AB was found to be active and AB derivatives such as 3-
methoxy-AB and orthoaminoazobenzene were far more active than the MAB-deriva-
tives (6, 9). Such discrepancy between carcinogenesis and mutagenesis is thought to
be due to a difference in the activation pathway. That is, the antibody to NADPH-
cytochrome P-450 reductase was found to inhibit the mutagenicities of azo dyes by
90% or more, indicating that the microsomal electron transport system participated
dominantly (11). Also, inhibition by the antibody to MC-P-448 was far larger (>90%)
than that by the antibody to the PB-P-450 (<20%). This shows that MC-P-448 is the

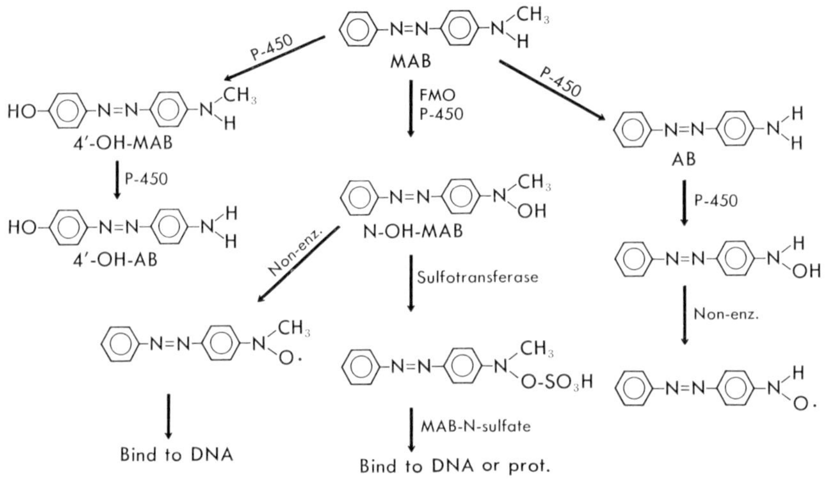

Fig. 10. Involvement of cytochrome P-450 system and FMO in the metabolism of MAB.

major component in mutagenic activation. These results can be reasonably explained by the fact that the AB derivatives, whose mutagenicities are extremely large, are metabolized exclusively by the cytochrome P-450 system (Fig. 10). In this sense, as far as aminoazo dyes are concerned, the activation pathway in mutagenesis is not necessarily the same as that in carcinogenic activation.

Naphthylamines

Naphthylamines have attracted special attention because of their carcinogenicity in man and numerous data on the metabolism of these compounds have been accumulated (1, 7, 13, 17, 40). As a result, it has become clear that the metabolic pathway leading to the active metabolite involves N-hydroxylation, as was true of the aminoazo dyes (13, 40). However, two important problems are still unsolved. The first is that two closely similar isomers of the naphthylamines are quite different in their carcinogenicity: 2-NA is strongly carcinogenic to bladder but 1-NA is completely non-carcinogenic (39, 42). The second problem is the kind of enzymes involved in the metabolism of napthylamines. These problems were studied from the standpoint of free radical formation.

1. Different features in free radical formation from 2-NA and 1-NA

2-NA and 1-NA were found to be metabolized by rat liver microsomes to give free radicals, but their features in free radical formation were different in two ways (35). Firstly, a large difference was observed between them in the production of free radicals: the former gave a large signal with distinct hyperfine structure, whereas the latter gave a far smaller signal without apparent hyperfine structure (Fig. 11). Secondly, when 2-NA was incubated with PB- or MC-microsomes, far larger ESR signals than with untreated microsomes appeared, whereas for 1-NA increases in the ESR signal with PB- or MC-microsomes were negligible (Fig. 11 a–d; Table II). As in the case of

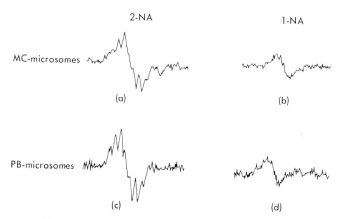

FIG. 11.   ESR signals of the free radicals produced by incubating 2-NA and 1-NA with MC- and PB-microsomes.

TABLE II.   Amounts of Free Radical Formed by Incubating 2-NA or 1-NA with Liver Microsomes from Non-treated, PB-treated, and MC-treated Rats[a]

Substrate	Microsomes		
	Non-treated	PB-treated	MC-treated
2-NA	0.105±0.011	0.264±0.065	0.251±0.042
1-NA	0.069±0.011	0.098±0.008	0.099±0.0026

[a] The amounts of free radical is given by the signal height/Mn^{2+}.

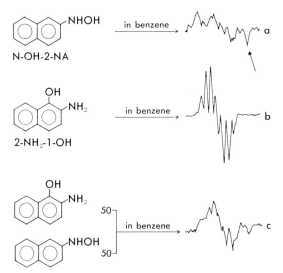

FIG. 12.   ESR signals of (a) authentic N-OH-2-NA, (b) authentic 2-amino-1-naphthol (2-NH$_2$-1-OH), and (c) mixture of equal molar concentrations of N-OH-2-NA and 2-NH$_2$-1-OH.

aminoazo dyes, free radicals were thought to be produced from enzymatically formed active metabolites. In the metabolism of 2-NA, the active metabolites, N-OH-2-NA and 2-amino-1-naphthol, have been identified (1). These two compounds are extremely reactive and quite easily convert autooxidatively into the corresponding free radicals, the ESR signals of which are indicated in Fig. 12a, b. None of these signals coincides with that observed by incubating 2-NA with microsomes. But the signal of the mixture containing equal molar concentrations of N-OH-2-NA and 2-amino-1-naphthol (Fig. 12c) coincided with the ESR signal obtained with MC-microsomes (Fig. 11a). It is significant that the ESR signal obtained by incubating 2-NA with PB-microsomes is different from that obtained with MC-microsomes: In the MC-microsomes, a trough due to the N-OH-2-NA radical is observed at the right-hand side (shown by arrow, Fig. 12a), whereas no such trough is observed in PB-microsomes. From these results, it is concluded that both N-OH-2-NA and 2-amino-1-naphthol are formed in the MC-microsomes, whereas with PB-microsomes the formation of the former metabolite was negligible. The relative importance in carcinogenesis of N-OH-2-NA and 2-amino-1-naphthol has been a subject of debate in naphthylamine carcinogenesis (1). However, recent studies have suggested that the N-hydroxylation is the activation pathway leading to tumorigenesis (13, 40). Thus, N-OH-2-NA binds covalently with DNA *in vitro* and its adducts were proved to be the same as those obtained from hepatic and urothelial DNA after administration of 2-NA to dogs (12, 16). Furthermore, urothelial tumors were induced by instilling N-OH-2-NA into the urinary bladder of dogs, and their incidence was greater than with its parent compound, 2-NA (41). In agreement with this, the nitroxide radical of N-OH-2-NA binds covalently with DNA (Fig. 13 a). From these facts, it appears that metabolic activation leading to N-OH-2-NA is more intimately correlated with the carcinogenesis process of 2-NA. However, this does not necessarily exclude 2-amino-1-naphthol from the active metabolites of 2-NA, since this metabolite was found to be carcinogenic, although its carcinogenicity is not potent (3). Binding of this metabolite was not so definite as the case of N-OH-2-NA; thus, its binding was proved by radioisotopic method (45), however, no free radical bound to DNA could be detected. When poly G was used instead of DNA, a bound radical could be detected (Fig. 13 b).

As indicated in Table II and Fig. 11, the amount of free radical formed by incubating 1-NA with MC- or PB-microsomes was much less than that from 2-NA. Its signal pattern and line width resemble those of an authentic sample of 1-amino-2-naphthol, while they are quite different from the signal pattern of authentic N OH-1-NA (Fig. 14). N-OH-1-NA is carcinogenic (2, 7, 41) and is considered to be the proximate form of 1-NA. Therefore, it is not premature to correlate the non-carcino-

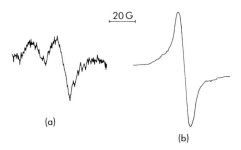

Fig. 13.   ESR signals of the covalently bound adducts of (a) N-OH-2-NA with DNA and (b) 2-amino-1-naphthol with poly G.

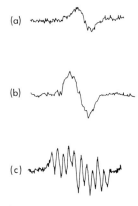

FIG. 14. ESR signals of (a) the free radical produced by incubating 1-NA with MC-microsomes, (b) authentic 1-amino-2-naphthol in benzene, (c) authentic N-OH-1-NA in benzene. Modulation amplitude: (a) 5.0 Gauss, (b) and (c) 3.2 Gauss.

genicity of 1-NA with the fact that nitroxide radical formation from this substance is far less than that from 2-NA.

2. Enzymes involved in the metabolism of naphthylamines

Poulsen *et al.* demonstrated that FMO participated in the N-hydroxylation of 2-NA. However, they did not describe the participation of the cytochrome P-450 enzyme system (*38*). Kawajiri *et al.*, on the other hand, reported that the mutagenicity of 2-NA was inhibited by the addition of antibodies against cytochromes P-448 and P-450 to the reaction mixture, and the inhibitory effect of the P-448 was found to be larger than that of P-450 (*18*). In the present ESR study, carbon monoxide inhibited the hydroxylation of 2-NA; thus, when the ratios of carbon monoxide and air were 1:1 and 19:1, the amount of free radical formed by MC-microsomes decreased by 25% and 42%, respectively, whereas the amount of free radical formed with PB-microsomes was decreased by 50% in both cases (*35*). These results show that the cytochrome P-450 system participated in the hydroxylation of 2-NA. The inhibitory effect was slightly larger in PB-microsomes than in MC-microsomes, indicating that 2-amino-1-naphthol is more sensitive to carbon monoxide than N-OH-2-NA. SKF-525A, an efficient inhibitor of the cytochrome P-450 system, inhibited the formation of the free radical in PB- and MC-microsomes to nearly the same degree: 35% and 32%, respectively (Fig. 15). The inhibitory effect of α-naphthoflavone, an inhibitor of cytochrome P-448, was somewhat different from that of SKF-525A: It inhibited the free radical formation in MC-microsomes (40%), whereas no inhibitory effect was observed in PB-microsomes (Fig. 15). From this it can be said that both cytochromes P-450 and P-448 are involved in the metabolic pathway leading to free radical formation. Further, the free radical formation was inhibited by 1-(1-naphthyl)-2-thiourea to the same extent (47% and 42%, respectively) in MC- and PB-microsomes (Fig. 15). This shows that FMO is also involved in the free radical formation. All the above evidence suggests that N-hydroxylation is catalyzed by both cytochrome P-448 and FMO, and this is analogous to the N-hydroxylation reaction of aminoazo dyes.

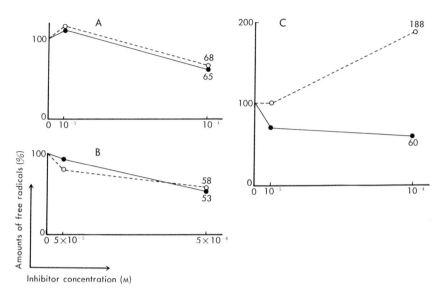

FIG. 15. Effects of SKF-525A (A), ANTU (B), and α-naphthoflavone (C) on the free radical formation from 2-NA. The amounts of free radical in the absence of the inhibitors is taken as 100.

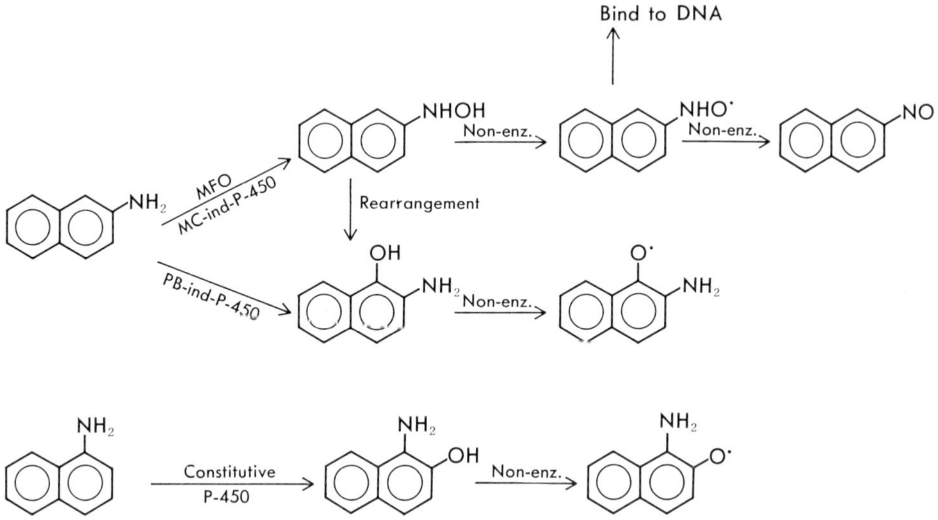

FIG. 16. Metabolic pathways of 2-NA and 1-NA and involvement of metabolizing enzymes.

The effects of enzyme inhibitors on the free radical formation could not be measured for 1-NA due to the small ESR signals observed (*35*). Therefore, the enzyme involved in the metabolism of 1-NA was difficult to determine. As seen in Table II, increase in enzyme activity in PB- and MC-induction are negligible. This is quite different from 2-NA where the free radical formation was significantly increased with MC- and PB-induction. The convertibility of the active metabolites of 2-NA and 1-NA into free radicals in organic solvents or in buffer solution is the same. Therefore, the difference between 2-NA and 1-NA in convertibility into free radicals is not the cause of the different amounts of free radicals produced. Alternatively, the following reasons may be considered: 1) The MC- and PB-induced cytochrome P-450 systems are involved in the metabolism of 2-NA but not in the metabolism of 1-NA. 2) The free radical formed from 1-NA is much more sensitive than that from 2-NA to scavenging by the metabolizing enzymes induced by MC and PB. Notwithstanding, in the metabolism of 1-NA, not the MC- and PB-induced cytochrome P-450 but the constitutive cytochrome P-450 system is thought to be mainly involved. From the above results, the enzymes involved in the metabolism of naphthylamines are considered to be as in Fig. 16. As seen, the metabolic pattern of carcinogenic 2-NA is quite different from that of the non-carcinogenic 1-NA. Such differences in the metabolism and free radical formation are thought to be the reason why 2-NA is carcinogenic and 1-NA is not.

Generation of Active Oxygens from the Active Forms of Aminoazo Dyes and Naphthylamines

In company with free radical formation from the active forms of aminoazo dyes and naphthylamines, active oxygens such as hydrogen peroxide and superoxide anion radical were generated in neutral buffer, as detected by the titanium sulfate method and nitro blue tetrazolium method, respectively (*36*). Good parallelism was found between the active oxygen formation and the convertibility to the free radical, and of especial interest is that the parallelism also extends to the carcinogenic activity of these compounds (Table III). Such a relation between the carcinogenic activity and the formation of free radical and active oxygens was observed previously for benzo[a]pyrene. Thus, this potent carcinogen was found to be converted enzymatically into the 6-oxy-

TABLE III. Generation of H_2O_2 and O_2^{-} from Active Metabolites of Naphthylamines and Aminoazo Dyes in Comparison with Their Carcinogenicity (at the Site of Administration) and Convertibility to the Free Radical

Compound	H_2O_2	O_2^{-}	Convertibility to the free radical	Carcino-genicity
N-OH-AB	+	+	+	+
N-OH-MAB	+	+	+	+
N-OH-1-NA	+	+	+	+
N-OH-2-NA	+	+	+	+
2-Amino-1-naphthol	+	+	+	+
1-Amino-2-naphthol	+	+	+	+
1-Amino-4-naphthol	+	+	+	−
1-Nitrosonaphthalene	−	−	+	±
2-Nitrosonaphthalene	−	−	+	±
1-Amino-5-naphthol	−	−	−	−
1-Amino-6-naphthol	−	−	−	−
1-Amino-7-naphthol	−	−	−	−
2-Amino-3-naphthol	−	−	−	−
1-NA	−	−	−	−
2-NA	−	−	−	−
1-Naphthol	−	−	−	−
2-Naphthol	−	−	−	−

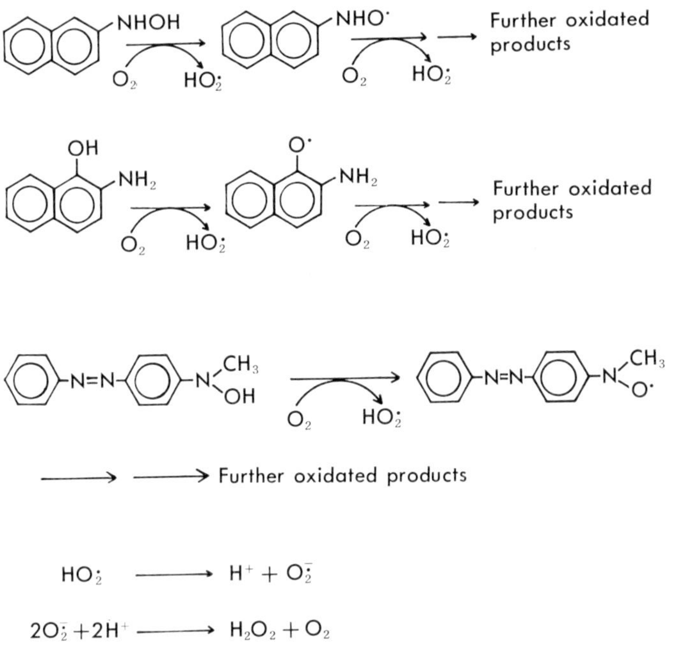

FIG. 17. Proposed scheme for the formation of hydrogen peroxide and super-oxide anion radical from N-OH-2-NA, 2-amino-1-naphthol, and N-OH-MAB.

benzo[a]pyrene radical (*30, 32, 34*), and at the same time the oxygen radical was generated (*25*). These findings seem to shed light on the unresolved problem in benzo[a]-pyrene carcinogenesis that benzo[a]pyrene-7,8-diol-9,10-epoxide, which has a significant ability to bind covalently to DNA, is not carcinogenic without application of a promoter such as TPA (*26*). This suggests that binding of the carcinogen to DNA alone is not sufficient to produce a tumor, but that cocarcinogenic and/or the promoting actions of some species is necessary. The most probable candidate for such a species is the concomitantly generated active oxygens. And the potent carcinogenicity of benzo[a]pyrene can be explained only when such a cooperative reaction of active metabolites and active oxygens is taken into account. The same relationship is considered true for aminoazo dyes and naphthylamines. That is, the free radical and active oxygens are formed concomitantly (Fig. 17), and cooperative actions of the binding of the active forms on one hand and the generation of active oxygens on the other hand is considered crucial for carcinogenicity. The intimate correlation among free radical formation, generation of active oxygens and carcinogenic activity in Table III may lend support to this proposition. Actually, this proposition is not unreasonable in view of the recent findings that active oxygens are extremely important in carcinogenesis, especially in cocarcinogenic and promoting actions (*5, 10, 19*).

Acknowledgment

This work was supported in part by a Grant-in-Aid from the Ministry of Education, Science and Culture of Japan.

REFERENCES

1. Arcos, J. C. and Argus, M. F. "Chemical Induction of Cancer," Vol. II B, pp. 217–301 (1974). Academic Press, New York.

2. Belman, S., Troll, W., Teebor, G., and Mukai, F. The carcinogenic and mutagenic properties of N-hydroxy-aminonaphthalenes. *Cancer Res.*, **28**, 535–542 (1968).

3. Bonser, G. M., Bradshaw, L., Clayson, D. B., and Jull, L. W. A further study of the carcinogenic properties of orthohydroxyamines and related compounds by bladder implantation in the mouse. *Br. J. Cancer*, **10**, 539–546 (1956).

4. Cook, J. W., Hewett, C. L., and Hieger, I. Isolation of a cancer-producing hydrocarbon from coal tar. II. Isolation of 1,2- and 4,5-benzopyrenes, perylene and 1, 2-benzanthracene. *J. Chem. Soc.*, 396–398 (1933).

5. Copeland, E. S. A National Institutes of Health Workshop report, Free radicals in promotion—A chemical pathway study section workshop. *Cancer Res.*, **43**, 5631–5637 (1983).

6. Degawa, M., Shoji, Y., Masuko, K., and Hashimoto, Y. Mutagenicity of metabolites of carcinogenic aminoazo dyes. *Cancer Lett.*, **8**, 71–76 (1979).

7. Deichmann, W. B. and Radomski, J. L. Carcinogenicity and metabolism of aromatic amines in the dog. *J. Natl. Cancer Inst.*, **43**, 263–269 (1969).

8. Guengerich, F. P. Separation and purification of multiple forms of microsomal cytochrome P-450. *J. Biol. Chem.*, **252**, 3970–3979 (1977).

9. Hashimoto, Y., Watanabe, H. K., and Degawa, M. Mutagenicity of 4-aminoazobenzene, N-hydroxy-4-aminoazobenzene, 4-nitrosoazobenzene, 4-nitroazobenzene, and their ring methoxylated derivatives on *Salmonella*. *Gann*, **72**, 921–929 (1981).

10. Hirota, N. and Yokoyama, T. Enhancing effect of hydrogen peroxide upon duodenal and upper jejunal carcinogenesis in rats. *Gann*, **72**, 811–812 (1981).

11. Igarashi, S., Yonekawa, H., Kawajiri, K., Watanabe, J., Kimura, T., Kodama, M., Nagata, C., and Tagashira, Y. Participation of the microsomal electron transport system in mutagenic activation of 4-dimethylaminoazobenzene, 4-methylaminoazobenzene and their 3′-methyl-derivatives. *Biochem. Biophys. Res. Commun.*, **106**, 164–169 (1982).

12. Kadlubar, F. F., Anson, J. F., Dooley, K. L., and Beland, F. A. Formation of urothelial and hepatic DNA adducts from the carcinogen 2-naphthylamine. *Carcinogenesis*, **2**, 467–470 (1981).

13. Kadlubar, F. F., Miller, J. A., and Miller, E. C. Hepatic microsomal N-glucuronidation and nucleic acid binding of N-hydroxy arylamines in relation to urinary bladder carcinogenesis. *Cancer Res.*, **37**, 805–814 (1977).

14. Kadlubar, F. F., Miller, J. A., and Miller, E. C. Microsomal N-oxidation of the hepatocarcinogen N-methyl-4-aminoazobenzene and the reactivity of N-hydroxy-N-methyl-4-aminoazobenzene. *Cancer Res.*, **36**, 1196–1206 (1976).

15. Kadlubar, F. F., Miller, J. A., and Miller, E. C. Hepatic metabolism of N-hydroxy-N-methyl-4-aminoazobenzene and other N-hydroxy arylamines to reactive sulfuric acid esters. *Cancer Res.*, **36**, 2350–2359 (1976).

16. Kadlubar, F. F., Unruh, L. E., Beland, F. A., Straub, K. M., and Evans, F. E. *In vitro* reaction of the carcinogen, N-hydroxy-2-naphthylamine, with DNA at the C-8 and N^2 atoms of guanine and at the N^6 atom of adenine. *Carcinogenesis*, **1**, 139–150 (1980).

17. Kadlubar, F. F., Unruh, L. E., Flammang, T. J., Sparks, D., Mitchum, R. K., and Mulder, G. J. Alteration of urinary levels of the carcinogen, N-hydroxy-2-naphthylamine, and its N-glucuronide in the rat by control of urinary pH, inhibition of metabolism of metabolic sulfation, and changes in biliary excretion. *Chem.-Biol. Interact.*, **33**, 129–147 (1981).

18. Kawajiri, K., Yonekawa, H., Harada, N., Noshiro, M., Omura, T., and Tagashira, Y. Immunochemical study on the role of different types of microsomal cytochrome P-450 in mutagenesis by chemical carcinogens. *Cancer Res.*, **40**, 1652–1657 (1980).

19. Kensler, T. W., Bush, D. M., and Kozumbo, W. J. Inhibition of tumor promotion by a biomimetic superoxide dismutase. *Science*, **221**, 75–77 (1983).

20. Kimura, T., Kodama, M., and Nagata, C. Nitroxide radicals generated from carcinogenic aminoazo dyes during their metabolism *in vivo* and in enzymatic system *in vitro*. *Biochem. Pharmacol.*, **28**, 557–560 (1979).

21. Kimura, T., Kodama, M., and Nagata, C. A correlation of the rate of N-hydroxylation of aminoazo dyes with their carcinogenic activity in the rat. *Carcinogenesis*, **3**, 1393–1396 (1982).

22. Kimura, T., Kodama, M., and Nagata, C. N-hydroxylation enzymes of carcinogenic aminoazo dyes: Possible involvement of cytochrome P-448. *Gann*, **73**, 55–62 (1982).

23. Kimura, T., Kodama, M., and Nagata, C. Purification of mixed function amine oxidase from rat liver microsomes. *Biochem. Biophys. Res. Commun.*, **110**, 640–645 (1983).

24. Kodama, M., Ioki, Y., and Nagata, C. Binding of benzo(a)pyrene-semiquinone radicals with DNA and polynucleotides. *Gann*, **68**, 253–254 (1977).

25. Lesko, S. A., Lorentzen, R. J., and Ts'o, P.O.P. Benzo(a)pyrene metabolism. One-electron pathways and the role of nuclear enzymes. *In* "Polycyclic Hydrocarbons and Cancer," ed. H. V. Gelboin and P.O.P. Ts'o, Vol. 1, pp. 261–269 (1978). Academic Press, New York.

26. Levin, W., Wood, A. W., Wislocki, P. G., Chang, R. L., Kapitulnik, J., Mah, H. D., Yagi, H., Jerina, D. M., and Conney, A. H. *In* "Polycyclic Hydrocarbons and Cancer," ed. H. V. Gelboin and P.O.P. Ts'o, Vol. 1, pp. 189–202 (1978). Academic Press, New York.

27. Matsushima, T., Grantham, P. H., Weisburger, E. K., and Weisburger, J. H. Phenobarbital-mediated increase in ring- and N-hydroxylation of the carcinogen N-2-fluorenylacetamid, and decrease in amounts bound to liver deoxyribonucleic acid. *Biochem. Pharmacol.*, **21**, 2043–2051 (1972).

28. Miller, J. A. Carcinogenesis by chemicals: An overview-G.H.A. Clowes memorial lecture. *Cancer Res.*, **30**, 559–576 (1970).

29. Miller, J. A. and Miller, E. C. The carcinogenic aminoazo dyes. *Adv. Cancer Res.*, **1**, 339–396 (1953).

30. Nagata, C., Inomata, M., Kodama, M., and Tagashira, Y. Electron spin resonance study on the interaction between the chemical carcinogens and tissue components. III. Determination of the structure of the free radical produced either by stirring 3, 4-benzopyrene with albumin or incubating it with liver homogenates. *Gann*, **59**, 289–298 (1968).

31. Nagata, C., Kodama, M., and Ioki, Y. Electron spin resonance study of the binding of the 6-oxybenzo(a)pyrene radical and benzo(a)pyrene-semiquinone radicals with DNA and polynucleotides. *In* "Polycyclic Hydrocarbons and Cancer," ed. H. V. Gelboin and P.O.P. Ts'o, pp. 247–260 (1978). Academic Press, New York.

32. Nagata, C., Kodama, M., Ioki, Y., and Kimura, T. Free radicals produced from chemical carcinogens and their significance in carcinogenesis. *In* "Free Radicals and Cancer," ed. R. A. Floyd, pp. 1–62 (1982). Marcel Dekker, New York.

33. Nagata, C., Kodama, M., Kimura, T., and Aida, M. Metabolically generated free radicals from many types of chemical carcinogens and binding of the radicals with nucleic acid bases. *In* "Carcinogenesis: Fundamental Mechanisms and Environmental Effects," ed. B. Pullman, P.O.P. Ts'o, and H. V. Gelboin, pp. 43–54 (1980). D. Reidel Publishing Company, Dordrecht.

34. Nagata, C., Tagashira, Y., and Kodama, M. Metabolic activation of benzo(a)pyrene:

Significance of the free radical. *In* "Chemical Carcinogenesis," ed. P.O.P. Ts'o and J. A. DiPaolo, pp. 87–111 (1974). Marcel Dekker, New York.

35. Nakayama, T., Kimura, T., Kodama, M., and Nagata, C. Electron spin resonance study on the metabolism of 2-naphthylamine and 1-naphthylamine in rat liver microsomes. *Gann*, **73**, 382–390 (1982).

36. Nakayama, T., Kimura, T., Kodama, M., and Nagata, C. Generation of hydrogen peroxide and superoxide anion from active metabolites of naphthylamines and aminoazo dyes: its possible role in carcinogenesis. *Carcinogenesis*, **4**, 765–769 (1983).

37. Patrianakos, C. and Hoffmann, D. Chemical studies on tobacco smoke. LXIV. On the analysis of aromatic amines in cigarette smoke. *J. Anal. Toxicol.*, **3**, 150–154 (1979).

38. Poulsen, L. L., Masters, B.S.S., and Ziegler, D. M. Mechanism of 2-naphthylamine oxidation catalyzed by pig liver microsomes. *Xenobiotica*, **6**, 481–498 (1976).

39. Purchase, L.F.H., Kalinowski, A. E., Ishmael, J., Wilson, J., Gore, C. W., and Chart, I. S. Lifetime carcinogenicity study of 1- and 2-naphthylamine in dogs. *Br. J. Cancer*, **44**, 892–901 (1981).

40. Radomski, J. L. and Brill, E. Bladder cancer induction by aromatic amines: Role of N-hydroxy metabolites. *Science*, **167**, 992–993 (1970).

41. Radomski, J. L., Brill, E., Deichmann, W. B., and Glass, E. M. Carcinogenicity testing of N-hydroxy and other oxidation and decomposition products of 1- and 2-naphthylamine. *Cancer Res.*, **31**, 1461–1467 (1971).

42. Radomski, J. L., Deichmann, W. B., Altman, N. H., and Radomski, T. Failure of pure 1-naphthylamine to induce bladder tumors in dogs. *Cancer Res.*, **40**, 3537–3539 (1980).

43. Thorgeirsson, S. S., Jollow, D. J., Sasame, H. A., Green, I., and Mitchel, J. R. The role of cytochrome P-450 in N-hydroxylation of 2-acetylaminofluorene. *Mol. Pharmacol.*, **9**, 398–404 (1973).

44. Thorgeirsson, S. S. and Nebert, D. W. The *Ah* locus and the metabolism of chemical carcinogens and other foreign compounds. *Adv. Cancer Res.*, **25**, 149–193 (1977).

45. Troll, W., Belman, S., and Levine, E. The effect of metabolites of 2-naphthylamine and the mutagen hydroxylamine on the thermal stability of DNA and polynucleotides. *Cancer Res.*, **23**, 841–847 (1963).

46. Welch, R. M., Gommi, B., Alvares, A. P., and Conney, A. H. Effect of enzyme induction on the metabolism of benzo[a]pyrene and 3'-methyl-4-monomethylaminoazobenzene in the pregnant and fetal rats. *Cancer Res.*, **32**, 973–978 (1972).

47. Wynder, E. L. and Goldsmith, R. The epidemiology of bladder cancer. *Cancer*, **40**, 1246–1268 (1977).

48. Yamagiwa, K., and Ichikawa, K. Pathogenesis of carcinoma. *Gann*, **12**, 1–29 (1918).

49. Ziegler, D. M., McKee, E. M., and Poulsen, L. L. Microsomal flavoprotein-catalyzed N-oxidation of arylamines. *Drug Metab. Dispos.*, **1**, 314–321 (1973).

MECHANISM OF METABOLIC ACTIVATION OF AFLATOXIN B₁

Yoshio Ueno, Fumio Tashiro, and Hiroko Nakaki

*Department of Toxicology and Microbial Chemistry, Faculty of Pharmaceutical Sciences, Tokyo University of Science**

Aflatoxin B_1 (AFB$_1$) is a naturally occurring carcinogen in food. Its potential for causing liver cancer in exposed human populations has been of great concern. This mycotoxin is activated into DNA-binding form(s) by the nuclear and microsomal cytochrome P-450 system of rat livers, and their activation potential is enhanced by pretreatment of animals with phenobarbital (PB) and polychlorinated biphenyl. Experiments with purified cytochrome P-450s revealed that P-450 I-a, one of the P-450 type partially purified from PCB-treated rates, possesses a high potential for activation of AFB$_1$, and this epoxidation process is regulated by cytochrome b_5. Conversion of AFB$_1$ into AFM$_1$, a much less active genotoxicant, is selectively mediated by P-448 II-a (high spin form); AFQ$_1$ formation is catalyzed by both types of P-450 and P-448. The existence of a cytosolic AFB$_1$-receptor is not demonstrated, but the specific interaction between "activated AFB$_1$" and "specific nuclear binding sites for glucocorticoid-receptor complex" is suggested.

Harmful effects of environmental agents on human health are currently a topic of great concern. Toxic fungal metabolites, so-called "mycotoxins," are naturally occurring pollutants in food and feed. Their possible long-term effects as carcinogens, mutagens, and teratogens have attracted the attention of health scientists.

Aflatoxin B_1 is one of the dihydrobisfuranoids produced by *Aspergillus flavus* and is a potent carcinogen in experimental animals. Several epidemiological surveys (*2, 3*) revealed a strong correlation between the uptake of AFB$_1$ and development of liver cancer.

As established in the literature, many enzymatic reactions are involved in carcinogenesis induced by chemical carcinogens. However, there is some discrepancy between data obtained *in vivo* and *in vitro*. *In vitro* experiments of AFB$_1$ revealed that the activation process, *i.e.*, the binding to DNA, is enhanced by the microsomal and nuclear fractions isolated from polychlorinated biphenyl (PCB)-treated rat liver (*8*). Conversely, a reduction of carcinogenic effect of AFB$_1$ was observed in phenobarbital (PB)-treated rats (*15*). The reduction of AFB$_1$-binding to rat liver macromolecules by PB-pretreatment *in vivo* was also observed (*7*).

In order to solve the problems of this discrepancy and elucidate the molecular mechanism of AFB$_1$ activation and metabolism, detailed experiments with nuclei,

TABLE I.   Mutagenicity of AFB$_1$ and Related Bisfuranoids

A :   *Rec* assay with *B. subtilis* (*21*)

Test compounds	μg/disc	Inhibition zone (mm)		*Rec* effect
		H17	M45	
AFB$_1$	20	0	10.0	++
AFB$_2$	100	0	0	—
AFG$_1$	100	0	7.5	+
AFG$_2$	100	0	0	—
Sterigmatocystin	1	0	2	+
	10	0	0	—

B :   Ames test with *S. typhimurium* TA98 (*22*)

Test compounds	μg/plate	Revertants/plate		Mutagenicity
		S-9 (−)	S-9 (+)	
AFB$_1$	0	30	20	
	0.01	29	323	+
	0.1	30	530	+
AFG$_1$	1	35	391	+
	10	34	369	+
Sterigmatocystin	1	28	133	+
	10	56	310	+

C :   Mammalian cell test with Chinese hamster cells (*16*)

Test compound	μg/ml	Induced mutation frequency/10^5 survivors		Mutagenicity
		S-9 (−)	S-9 (+, 1%)	
Sterigmatocystin	0	0	0	
	0.1	0	5.0	+
	0.2	0	26.0	+
	0.5	0	360.0	+

microsomes, and purified cytochrome P-450s were performed; some factors that modify aflatoxin metabolism were analyzed.

Genotoxicity of Aflatoxin B$_1$ (AFB$_1$)

In order to elucidate the molecular mechanism of the AFB$_1$ activation process, the genotoxicity of AFB$_1$ was evaluated by employing microbial and mammalian test systems. In *Rec* assay (*21*) with recombination-deficient mutant cells of *Bacillus subtilis*, AFB$_1$ and related mycotoxins such as AFG$_1$ and sterigmatocystin were shown to possess DNA-attacking ability, as summarized in Table I. However, AFB$_2$ and AFG$_2$ reacted negatively in this test assay. Since AFB$_2$ and AFG$_2$ lack the terminal double bond in bisfuran ring, this double bond seems important for their DNA-attacking ability, as has been discussed in previous reports. Further experiments with the Ames test revealed mutagenic activity of AFB$_1$, AFG$_1$, and sterigmatocystin in the presence of S-9 fraction of rat liver (Table I) (*22*). Mammalian cell culture tests also proved that sterigmatocystin, a potent carcinogen (*10*), produces a high level of mutation frequency in

Chinese hamster cells only when the liver activation system is present (16). The structure of sterigmatocystin also contains a dihydrobisfuran ring.

These experiments confirmed that AFB$_1$ and related dihydrobisfuranoid mycotoxins are potent mutagens in microbial and mammalian cells. Their genotoxic activities are induced by the biotransforming potential of the hepatic activation system.

Nuclear Activation of Aflatoxin B$_1$

Carcinogenic polycyclic hydrocarbons such as benzo[a]pyrene are also believed to require metabolic activation prior to tumor formation. These compounds are preferentially metabolized at the microsomal level by mixed function oxygenases. Recently, a similar enzyme system has been found in rodent liver nuclei. Vaught et al. (25) and Guengerich (8) investigated the metabolism of AFB$_1$ in hepatic nuclei of rats.

In our study (27), the nuclei were prepared from rats pretreated with PB, 3-methylcholanthrene (MC), and PCB, and their drug-metabolizing activities as well as the activation potential of AFB$_1$ were compared. As shown in Table II, aminopyrine-

TABLE II. Induction of Nuclear and Microsomal Drug-metabolizing Enzyme Activities in the Liver of Rats

Inducers	Fractions	Aminopyrine N-demethylase	Aniline hydroxylase	Epoxide hydrase
		(nmol products/mg protein/min)[a]		
—	Nuclei	0.21	0.05	0.42
	Microsomes	3.96	1.26	4.72
PB	Nuclei	0.46	0.06	0.97
	Microsomes	9.95	1.73	19.93
MC	Nuclei	0.15	0.07	0.59
	Microsomes	1.66	1.28	5.99
PCB	Nuclei	0.37	0.08	1.21
	Microsomes	7.47	2.14	27.78

[a] Means of 2 experiments each consisting of triple determinations.

TABLE III. Nuclear Activation of AFB$_1$

Inducers	Microsomes	[^{3}H]AFB$_1$ bound[a] (pmol/mg DNA)	Ratio
Control	—	270[b]	1[c]
	+	1,060	
PB	—	960	4
	+	2,040	
MC	—	300	1
	+	610	
PCB	—	1,040	4
	+	2,040	

[a] Nuclei isolated from the three pooled livers of rats, each untreated or pretreated with inducers, were incubated with 7×10^{-6} M [^{3}H]AFB$_1$ for 60 min, in the presence or absence of respective microsomes. A pair of nuclei and microsomes was isolated from the same liver specimen.

[b] Mean of two experiments each consisting of triple determinations.

[c] Ratio of AFB$_1$ activation of induced nuclei to that of control.

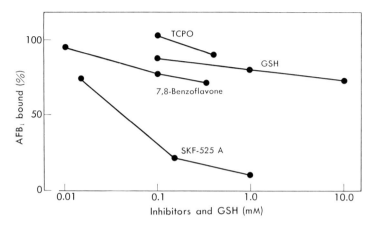

F<small>IG</small>. 1. Effects of metabolic inhibitors and glutathione (GSH) on the binding of AFB₁ to nuclear DNA. Nuclei isolated from PCB-treated rats were incubated with 7×10^{-5} M AFB₁ for 60 min. TPCO, 7,8-benzoflavone, and SKF-525A were dissolved in DMSO, and glutathione was dissolved in distilled water and adjusted to pH 7.4 prior to use. The final concentration of DMSO was adjusted to 1.2%. The activity was expressed as % of control.

N-demethylase, aniline hydroxylase, and epoxide hydrase were markedely increased both in the nuclei and microsomal fractions of rats pretreated with various drug-metabolizing inducers. These preparations were then used to test the nuclear activation of AFB₁ in the presence and absence of fortified microsomal systems. As shown in Table III, the nuclear activation of AFB₁ observed in the control was quadrupled by pretreatment with PB and PCB; no significant elevation was observed in the nuclei prepared from MC-treated rats. Furthermore, supplementation of respective microsomal fractions to the nuclear system enhanced the binding of AFB₁ to nuclear DNA.

In order to elucidate the possible participation of cytochrome P-450 system in the AFB₁-activation process, the effect of inhibitors of the cytochrome P-450 system were analyzed (Fig. 1) (23). The binding of AFB₁ to nuclear DNA was significantly inhibited by SKF-525A, a potent inhibitor of P-450 type; 7,8-benzoflavone, an inhibitor of P-448 type, was less effective. Our work with inducers and inhibitors revealed that activation of AFB₁ in DNA-binding form(s) is mediated by cytochrome P-450 type with the absorption peak at 450 nm in the carbon monoxide difference spectrum.

It is well known that AFB₁ is transformed into 8,9-epoxy AFB₁ and this active intermediate is presumed to bind guanine residue of DNA, though the intermediate is not chemically defined (5). Carcinogenic polycyclic hydrocarbons such as benzo[a]pyrene are also activated into epoxide derivatives and epoxide hydrase regulates the level of this active form. Therefore, we examined possible participation of this enzyme in the AFB₁ activation process in nuclear preparations by introducing trichloropropane oxide (TCPO), a potent inhibitor of epoxide hydrase. As shown in Figs. 1 and 2, AFB₁ binding to nuclear DNA was slightly depressed by 0.4 mM TCPO in the nuclei prepared from PCB-treated rats. In the reconstituted nuclear system composed of stripped nuclei with Triton X-100 and PCB-microsomes meanwhile, 0.1–0.4 mM TCPO markedly enhanced the amount of AFB₁ bound to nuclear DNA (23). It seems, therefore, that not only is AFB₁ activated into DNA-binding form(s) by microsomes, but also an inhibition

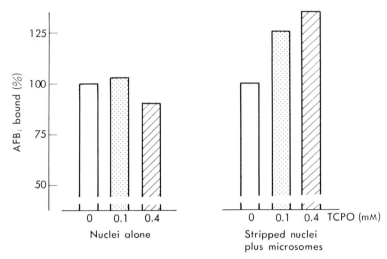

FIG. 2.   Effect of TCPO on the binding of AFB$_1$ to nuclear DNA. Intact nuclei isolated from PCB-treated rat liver or Triton X-100-treated nuclei (stripped nuclei) supplemented with PCB-microsomes (0.54 mg protein) was incubated with 7×10^{-5} M AFB$_1$ in the presence or absence of TCPO. TCPO was dissolved in DMSO, and the final concentration of DMSO was 0.8%. AFB$_1$ bound to nuclear DNA was expressed as % of control.

of epoxide hydrase by TCPO causes an increased amount of AFB$_1$ binding to nuclear DNA. From this we infer that the level of epoxide hydrase may regulate the nuclear binding of AFB$_1$.

Activation of Aflatoxin B_1 by Cytochrome P-450s

It has recently been shown that microsomal cytochrome P-450 is composed of multiple forms of isoenzymes. We, therefore, introduced a reconstituted cytochrome P-450 system for evaluation of its isoenzymes in xenobiotic metabolism. Its components were cytochrome P-450s, NADPH-cytochrome c reductase (fp$_T$), and phospholipids.

Thus, the metabolic functions of purified cytochrome P-450s from PB, MC, and PCB-treated rat livers were analyzed in regards to the activation and metabolism of AFB$_1$ (24, 28).

Table IV summarizes data of the major forms of cytochrome P-450s purified from PB- and MC-treated rat livers (28). PB-P-450 and MC-P-448 respectively purified from PB- and MC-treated rat livers, catalyzed the activation of AFB$_1$ into DNA binding form(s) in 17 and 11 pmol/nmol cytochrome/min, respectively. This means that the activation potential of the cytochrome P-450 type was only 50% greater than that of the P-448 type; no significant selectivity of the cytochrome P-450s towards the activation of AFB$_1$ was demonstrated.

Recently, a simple and reproducible method of separating multiple forms of cytochrome P-450s of PCB-treated rat livers was developed employing ω-amino-n-octyl Sepharose 4B and DE-cellulose column chromatographies (13). From the microsomes of PCB-treated rats, seven P-450 type cytochromes (I-a to I-g) and five P-448 types (II-a to II-e) were fractionated. Six of the 12 fractions were used to examine the selec-

TABLE IV. Metabolism and Activation of AFB_1 by PB-P-450 and MC-P-448
in Reconstituted Cytochrome P-450 System (28)

Cytochromes	AFM_1	AFQ_1	DNA-binding
		(pmol/nmol cytochrome/min)	
PB-P-450	0	0	17
MC-P-448	230	13	11

TABLE V. Activation of AFB_1 in the Reconstituted Cytochrome P-450
System and Enhancing Effect of Cytochrome b_5

Cytochrome P-450	[^{3}H]AFB_1 bound (pmol/nmol P-450/min)[a]	
	Minus cytochrome b_5	Plus cytochrome b_5[b]
P-450 type I-a	152.5	223.0 (143)[b]
I-c	5.5	12.5 (225)
I-d	13.0	28.6 (200)
P-448 type II-a	2.0	2.4 (120)
II-b	3.0	3.4 (113)
II-c	4.0	4.0 (100)

[a] An average of 2–3 determinations.
[b] An equimolar amount of cytochrome b (0.05 nmol) was supplemented. Parentheses indicate % of
the control.

TABLE VI. Drug-metabolizing Activities of Cytochrome P-450s Fractionated
from Hepatic Microsomes of PCB-treated Rats

Cytochrome P-450	Aminopyrine N-demethylase	Aniline hydroxylase	Dimethylaniline N-demethylase
		(nmol products/nmol P-450/min)[a]	
P-450 type I-a	3.8	2.04	26.1
I-c	4.1	2.09	19.7
I-d	4.6	2.54	5.0
P-448 type II-a	1.2	0.23	2.0
II-b	1.3	0.30	4.7
II-c	2.1	0.33	3.3

[a] All data are an average of two separate experiments with duplicate estimations.

tivity of cytochrome P-450s on the activation and metabolism of AFB_1 (24). The effect
on the activation of AFB_1 by cytochrome b_5, an important element in the microsomal
oxidation reaction, was also investigated. As summarized in Table V, in the absence of
cytochrome b_5 (0.05 nmol), the cytochrome P-450 I-a exhibited maximal binding
activity (152.5 nmol AFB_1 bound/pmol P-450/min). This is $9\times$ and $15\times$ greater than
the values obtained with the major forms of PB-P-450 and MC-P-448, respectively.
The binding activity of other P-450 types I-c and I-d were 5.5 and 13.0 pmol AFB_1
bound, respectively. These values are comparable to those obtained with the major
forms of PB- and MC-microsomes. On the contrary, the binding activity of P-448 types
(II-a, b, and c) were far less active. Interestingly, cytochrome b_5 has an enhancing
effect only in the binding of AFB_1 mediated by P-450 type cytochromes.

The drug-metabolizing activities of these fractions are summarized in Table VI.

TABLE VII. Effect of Anti P-450 I-a on PCB-microsomal Drug
Metabolism and Activation of AFB₁

Antibody	Aminopyrine N-demethylase (nmol/nmol P-450/min)	% of control	AFB₁ bound (nmol/nmol P-450/mg DNA/60 min)	% of control
Control	4.79	100	8.3	100
Anti I-a	3.42	71	5.0	60

Cytochrome P-450 type I-a possesses a high activity in dimethylaniline N-demethylase. Physicochemical analysis revealed that absorption maximum of P-450 I-a in a reduced carbon monoxide difference spectrum was 450.0 nm, and its yield was about 20–25% of the total PCB-P-450s.

In order to evaluate this unique P-450 I-a in PCB-microsomal activation of AFB₁, anti-P-450 I-a was prepared and added to the reaction system composed of PCB-microsomes, DNA, and [³H]AFB₁. The data indicated that the anti P-450 I-a decreased the DNA binding of AFB₁ to 60% of the control (Table VII). Judging from these immunological approaches, the P-450 I-a fraction is actually thought to play an important role in activation of AFB₁ in the PCB-microsomes.

Significance of Cytochrome b_5 in Aflatoxin B_1 Activation

As shown in Table V, the supplement of cytochrome b_5 stimulated the AFB₁-activation reaction. To clarify the optimal ratio of the concentration of cytochrome b_5 to cytochrome P-450, the activation of AFB₁ by the cytochrome fraction I-a was measured in the presence of various amounts of cytochrome b_5. Results revealed that maximal

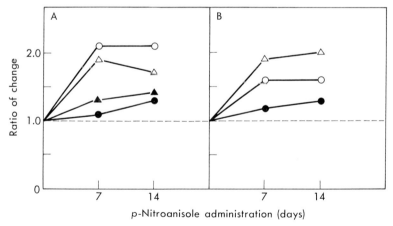

FIG. 3. Changes in the components of microsomal electron transport system and drug metabolizing activities in p-nitroanisole-treated rats. Male rats were daily administered with 250 mg/kg of p-nitroanisole orally for 7 and 14 days, and the microsomal components and their activities were expressed as the ratio to the control. A: relative ratio of components of electron transport system. ○ cytochrome b_5; △ fp_T; ▲ cytochrome P-450; ● NADH-cytochrome c reductase (fp_D). B: relative ratio of drug-metabolizing activities. △ p-nitroanisole; ○ aminopyrine; ● aniline.

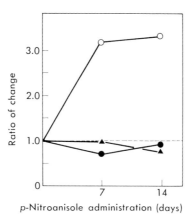

FIG. 4. Relative activity of microsomal activation and metabolism of AFB$_1$ in the liver of rats treated with p-nitroanisole. ○ AFB$_1$-DNA; ▲ AFM$_1$; ● AFQ$_1$.

binding (1.6× of the control) was observed with the ratio of 0.25 cytochrome b_5: 1.0 cytochrome P-450; the excess cytochrome b_5 depressed the AFB$_1$ binding to DNA (24).

Recent evidence has shown that during the enzymatic processes of microsomal drug oxidation, the first of two electrons required for cytochrome P-450-mediated oxidation is donated by NADPH or NADH *via* cytochrome b_5 (11). The participation of cytochrome b_5 in drug oxidation is demonstrated by the demethylation and hydroxylation reactions. Our present work indicates that activation of AFB$_1$, which is mediated by the epoxidation of a terminal double bond of bisfuran ring of AFB$_1$ (5), is also stimulated by cytochrome b_5.

According to Sugiyama *et al.* (19), the administration of p-nitroanisole to rats only induced cytochrome b_5 without an elevation of cytochrome P-450 level in the liver. Utilizing their procedure, we investigated the significance of cytochrome b_5 in the metabolic activation process of AFB$_1$.

As shown in Fig. 3, the daily administration of p-nitroanisole in doses of 250 mg/kg for 7 and 14 days caused a marked elevation of cytochrome b_5 content in hepatic microsomes. The levels of cytochrome P-450 and cytochrome c reductases were comparable with those of controls.

We used these microsomal preparations, rich in cytochrome b_5 content, to examine their potential for AFB$_1$ activation. The microsomes prepared from p-nitroanisole treated rats yielded a significantly high amount of DNA bound AFB$_1$ (Fig. 4). Therefore, it seems probable that the level of cytochrome b_5 may regulate the activation potential of microsomes toward AFB$_1$. Introduction of anti-cytochrome b_5 to the reaction system may validate this assumption. Furthermore, the possibility that p-nitroanisole induces a specific cytochrome P-450 with a high affinity to AFB$_1$ is not ruled out.

Hydroxylation of Aflatoxin B$_1$

Hydroxylation of bisfuran and cyclopentanone rings of AFB$_1$ results in the respective formation of AFM$_1$ and AFQ$_1$. O-Demethylation yields AFP$_1$, as shown in

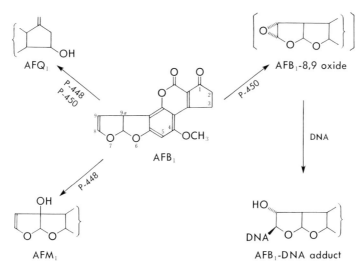

FIG. 5. Metabolic transformation of AFB₁.

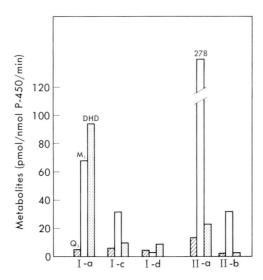

FIG. 6. Metabolism of AFB₁ in reconstituted cytochrome P-450 system of PCB-treated rats. AFB₁ was incubated with cytochrome P-450s fractionated from the livers of PCB-treated rats in the presence of fp_T, NADP, G-6-P, and others for 60 min, and the metabolites were estimated. ▨ AFQ₁; □ AFM₁; ▨ AFB₁-dihydrodiol (DHD).

Fig. 5. Therefore, we tried to determine if these hydroxylation and demethylation reactions of AFB₁ are catalyzed by specific cytochrome P-450s. As shown in Table IV, the major form of MC-microsomes (P-448) selectively catalyzed the formation of AFM₁ in the reconstituted cytochrome P-450 system, while the PB-P-450 catalyzed the formation of both AFM₁ and AFQ₁ (28). Recent experiments with PCB-P-450s revealed that, as summarized in Fig. 6, a marked formation of AFM₁ was observed with P-448 II-a (high-spin form). P-450 I-a also catalyzed the formation of AFM₁ but its potential

TABLE VIII. Relative Genotoxicity of Aflatoxins

Aflatoxins	Relative mutagenicity to *S. typhimurium* TA98 (%)	Relative carcinogenicity *via* 12 month dietary exposure
AFB$_1$	100.0[a]	Most potent hepatocarcinogen
Aflatoxicol	56.0	~50% as potent as AFB$_1$
AFG$_1$	5.5	Less potent than AFB$_1$
AFM$_1$	2.0	~30% as potent as AFB$_1$[b]
AFB$_2$	1.0	Non-tumorigenic
AFP$_1$	1.0	Not tested
AFQ$_1$	0.2	~100× less potent than AFB$_1$

[a] Ames test with PCB-microsomes as an activating system (*1, 22*).

[b] Carcinogenic potential of AFM$_1$ is presumed to be much less active than AFB$_1$, because Fisher rats developed hepatocellular carcinoma with 100% incidence 17 months after exposure to 50 ppb AFB$_1$, but no carcinoma were detected with 50 ppb AFM$_1$ (*12*).

was far less active than P-448 II-a. Other isoenzymes of cytochrome P-450s produced no significant amount of AFM$_1$.

As for AFQ$_1$, all isoenzymes examined produced this hydroxylated metabolite. Thus, specificity of cytochrome P-450s was not demonstrated. No precise information on the formation of AFP$_1$ is available because of the low-level production of this de-methylated product under the experimental conditions employed.

These metabolites are biologically much less active than AFB$_1$ and, as such, are considered to be detoxication products, in spite of Sinnhuber *et al.*'s report (*18*) that AFM$_1$ has some carcinogenic activity in rainbow trout. Aflatoxicol (AFL) is formed by a reduction mediated by cytosolic enzymes.

Since these metabolites exist in very small quantities, prudent methods are indicated to evaluate their toxicological activity. Wong and Hsieh (*26*) demonstrated good correlations between the relative mutagenic activity and *in vivo* carcinogenicity of AF metabolites, using the frame shift detector of *Salmonella typhimurium* TA 98 in conjunction with rat S-9 fraction. Coulombe *et al.* (*4*) demonstrated similar findings in the trout hepatic enzyme activation system. As shown in Table VIII, mutagenic activity of AFB$_1$ and its metabolites to *S. typhimurium* TA 98, in conjunction with the PCB-microsomal activation system, also demonstrated good correlation between *in vitro* and *in vivo* carcinogenicity tests.

Inactivation of Aflatoxin B$_1$ Activation by Thiols

As discussed above, the binding of AFB$_1$ to nuclear DNA is mediated *via* its epoxidation by cytochrome P-450s. However, this intermediate, AFB$_1$-8,9-oxide, is very unstable and reactive with nucleophilic compounds such as thiols. Lotlikar *et al.* (*14*) reported that microsome-mediated binding of AFB$_1$ to DNA was inhibited by a gluta-thione-S-transferase system localized in the hepatic cytosol of rats. Friedman *et al.* (*6*) also investigated the inactivation of AFB$_1$ mutagenicity by thiols. To confirm previous evidence, AFB$_1$ was incubated with PCB-nuclei in the presence of PCB-microsomes, and followed by estimation of AFB$_1$ bound to nuclear DNA. As shown in Table IX, of the four thiols tested, glutathione was the most active compound, reducing DNA

TABLE IX. Inhibitory Effect of Thiols on AFB₁ Binding to Nuclear DNA

Thiols (5 mM)	[³H]AFB₁ bound to DNA[a]	
	pmol/nmol P-450/min	Control (%)
—	85	100
Glutathione	35	41
Cysteine	80	94
Mercaptoethanol	82	95
Dithiothreitol	78	91

[a] Nuclei were incubated with [³H]AFB₁ in the presence of PCB-microsomes.

bound AFB₁ to 41% of the control value. This finding supports previous evidence that glutathione possesses a protective effect on AFB₁-induced mutagenicity and DNA-binding.

Cytosolic Receptor and Nuclear Acceptor of Aflatoxin B₁

Another important aspect of AFB₁ carcinogenicity is the immediate propensity of this potent carcinogen to liver nuclei. AFB₁ is either directly transported to hepatic nuclei, where the activation and DNA modification take place, or an unknown cytosolic receptor (or carrier factor) catalyzes its transport to the nuclei. In order to clarify this current problem, the possibility of the presence of a cytosolic receptor and nuclear acceptor of AFB₁ was investigated (20). Upon incubation of [³H]AFB₁ with the hepatic cytosol of Fisher rats, which are highly susceptible to AFB₁ carcinogenicity, dextrane-coated charcoal and sucrose gradient centrifugation methods were adopted for analysis of the formation of an AFB₁-receptor complex. However, all trials failed to demonstrate

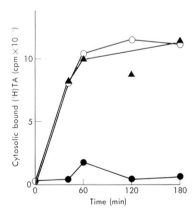

FIG. 7. Effect of AFB₁ on the formation of triamcinoline acetonide-cytosolic receptor complex. The hepatic cytosol 100 μl, [³H]TA 1.0 ng and ethanol 10 μl, in total volume of 110 μl, were incubated at 0° for desired times, and the reaction was stopped by an addition of 100 μl of dextrane-coated charcoal. After standing for 15 min and followed by centrifugation at 2,500 × g for 15 min, the radioactivity in the supernatant was estimated. ○ [³H]TA (2.3 pmol) alone; ▲ added with AFB₁ (3.2 nmol); ● added with cold TA (4.6 nmol).

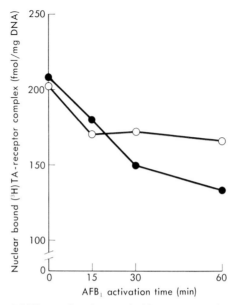

F<small>IG</small>. 8.   Effect of AFB$_1$ on the glucocorticoid receptor-nuclear binding. Potassium phosphate buffer (pH 7.4) 30 μmol, MgCl$_2$ 2.5 μmol, EDTA 0.2 μmol.
NADPH 0.75 μmol, PCB-microsomes 0.54 nmol P-450, and nuclei 0.67 mg DNA,
in total volume of 0.25 ml, were incubated at 20° for desired times in the absence
or presence of AFB$_1$ 75 nmol dissolved in DMSO. The reaction was stopped by an
addition of ice-cold 0.25 M sucrose-10 mM MgCl$_2$ (1 ml) and followed by centrifugation at 3,000 rpm for 15 min. The nuclear pellet, suspended in 200 μl of
0.25 M sucrose-10 mM MgCl$_2$, was added with 200 μl of "activated cytosol-[^{3}H]
TA complex" and followed by an incubation at 0° for 1 hr. The radioactivity
bound to the nuclei was estimated. ○ control nuclei; ● AFB$_1$-treated nuclei.

a cytosolic receptor for AFB$_1$. One trial with [^{3}H]triamcinolone acetonide (TA), a
synthetic glucocorticoid and a tool for researches on its receptor, is shown in Fig. 7.
This glucocorticoid binds with the hepatic cytosol to form a [^{3}H]TA-receptor complex
proportional to the incubation period. This complex formation was completely inhibited
by the addition of 2,000× the amount of cold TA; however, no inhibition was observed with about 1,500× AFB$_1$. This indicates that AFB$_1$ did not compete with TA
for the cytosolic TA receptor.

   In order to elucidate the possible interaction of AFB$_1$ with nuclear acceptor sites
for TA-receptor complex, the intact nuclei isolated from rat livers were incubated with
"activated" [^{3}H]TA-receptor complex bound to nuclei. Figure 8 shows that about
200 fmol of the complex were accepted by the nuclear DNA-acceptor region when the
nuclei were preincubated with dimethylsulfoxide (DMSO) (solvent control) and PCB-
microsomes. When the nuclei were preincubated with AFB$_1$ in the presence of PCB-
microsomes, followed by analysis of their potential for acceptance of the complex, the
nuclear transfer of the complex was decreased to 85 and 80% of the control after 30
and 60 min incubations, respectively.

   These data reveal that AFB$_1$ uptaken into the hepatic tissue was directly metabolized
into the active form by the microsomal cytochrome P-450 system. This active intermediate binds with nuclear regions that are identical to the acceptor site of the TA-

receptor complex, or a nearby specific site which regulates the binding of the TA-receptor complex to nuclear acceptors.

According to Pfahl (17), rat and mouse glucocorticoid receptors were found to interact with a high affinity site or sites in or near the promoter region of the mouse mammary tumor (MMTV) proviral DNA. Our present findings strongly suggest specific interactions between "activated AFB$_1$" and "DNA binding sites specific for glucocorticoid-receptor complexes".

This important new evidence of active AFB$_1$-DNA interaction strongly suggests further research to determine how genes are affected and the genetic expression is modified by the activation of chemical carcinogens.

Acknowledgments

This research was partly aided by a Cancer Research Grant from the Ministry of Education, Science and Culture, Japan. The authors thank Drs. R. Kato and T. Kamataki (Keio University School of Medicine) for supplying specimens of cytochrome P-450s. Technical assistance of Y. Mine, I. Sekiguchi, A. Tomioka, Y. Mabe, K. Onda, and Y. Emi was greatly appreciated. We also thank Dr. G. Naase (University of Maryland) for skillful assistance in preparation of the manuscript.

REFERENCES

1. Ames, B. N., Durston, W. E., Yamazaki, E., and Lee, F. D. Carcinogens are mutagens: A simple test system combining liver homogenates for activation and bacteria for detection. *Proc. Natl. Acad. Sci. U. S.*, **70**, 2281–2285 (1973).
2. Anukarahanonta, T. and Chudhalbuddhi, C. High-performance liquid chromatography of aflatoxins in human urine. *J. Chromatogr.*, **275**, 387–393 (1983).
3. Bulatao-Jayme, J., Almero, E. M., Castro, M.C.A., Jardeleza, M.T.R., and Salamat, L. A. A case-control dietary study of primary liver cancer risk from aflatoxin exposure. *Int. J. Epidemiol.*, **11**, 112–119 (1982).
4. Coulombe, R. A., Shelton, D. W., Sinnhuber, R. O., and Nixon, J. E. Comparative mutagenicity of aflatoxins using a *Salmonella*/trout hepatic enzyme activation system. *Carcinogenesis*, **3**, 1261–1264 (1982).
5. Essigman, J. M., Croy, R. G., Nadzan, A. M., Busby, Jr. W. F., Reinhold, V. N., Büchi, G., and Wogan, G. N. Structural identification of the major DNA adduct formed by aflatoxin B$_1$ *in vitro*. *Proc. Natl. Acad. Sci. U. S.*, **74**, 1870–1874 (1977).
6. Friedman, M., Wehr, C. M., Schade, J. E., and MacGregor, J. T. Inactivation of aflatoxin B$_1$ mutagenicity by thiols. *Fd Chem. Toxicol.*, **20**, 887–892 (1982).
7. Garner, R. C. Reduction in binding of [^{14}C]aflatoxin B$_1$ to rat liver macromolecules by phenobarbitone pretreatment. *Biochem. Pharmacol.*, **24**, 1553–1556 (1975).
8. Guengerich, F. P. Similarity of nuclear and microsomal cytochromes P-450 in the *in vitro* activation of aflatoxin B$_1$. *Biochem. Pharmacol.*, **28**, 2883–2890 (1979).
9. Gurtoo, H. L. and Dave, C. V. *In vitro* metabolic conversion of aflatoxins and benzo[a]-pyrene to nuclei acid-binding metabolites. *Cancer Res.*, **35**, 382–389 (1975).
10. Hendricks, J. D., Sinnhuber, R. O., Wales, J. H., Stack, M. E., and Hsieh, D.P.H. Hepatocarcinogenicity of sterigamatocystin and versicolorin A to rainbow trout (*Salmo gardneri*) embryos. *J. Natl. Cancer Inst.*, **64**, 1503–1509 (1980).
11. Hildebrandt, A. and Estabrook, R. W. Evidence for the participation of cytochrome b_5 in hepatic microsomal mixed-function oxidation reactions. *Arch. Biochem. Biophys.*, **143**, 66–79 (1971).

12. Hsieh, D.P.H. and Ruebner, B. H. An assessment of cancer risk from aflatoxins B_1 and M_1. *In* "Toxigenic Fungi: Their Toxins and Health Hazards," ed. H. Kurata and Y. Ueno, pp. 332–338 (1984). Elsevier, Amsterdam/Oxford, New York and Tokyo.

13. Kamataki, T., Maeda, K., Yamazoe, Y., Matsuda, N., Ishii, K., and Kato, R. A high-spin form of cytochrome P-450 highly purified from polychlorinated biphenyl-treated rats. *Mol. Pharmacol.*, **24**, 146–155 (1983).

14. Lotlikar, P. D., Insetta, S. M., Lyons, P. A., and Jhee, E.-C. *Cancer Lett.*, **8**, 143–149 (1980).

15. McLean, A.E.M. and Marshall, A. Reduced carcinogenic effects of aflatoxin in rat given phenobarbitone. *Br. J. Exp. Pathol.*, **52**, 322–329 (1971).

16. Noda, K., Umeda, M., and Ueno, Y. Cytotoxic and mutagenic effects of sterigmatocystin on cultured Chinese hamster cells. *Carcinogenesis*, **2**, 945–949 (1981).

17. Pfahl, M. Specific binding of the glucocorticoid-receptor complex to the mouses mammary tumor proviral promotor region. *Cell*, **31**, 475–482 (1982).

18. Sinnhuber, R. O., Lee, D. J., Wales, J. H., Landers, M. K., and Keyl, A. C. Hepatic carcinogenesis of aflatoxin M_1 in rainbow trout (*Salmo gardneri*) and its enhancement by cyclopropene fatty acids. *J. Natl. Cancer Inst.*, **53**, 1285–1288 (1974).

19. Sugiyama, T., Miki, N., and Yamano, T. NADH- and NADPH-dependent reconstituted *p*-nitroanisole *O*-demethylation system containing cytochrome P-450 with high affinity for cytochrome b_5. *J. Biochem.*, **87**, 1457–1467 (1980).

20. Tashiro, F., Emi, Y., and Ueno, Y. Effect of aflatoxin B_1 on the nuclear binding of triamcinolone-receptor complex in rat liver. Abstr. 104th Ann. Meet. Jpn. Pharm. Soc., p. 442 (1984).

21. Ueno, Y. and Kubota, K. DNA-attacking ability of carcinogenic mycotoxins in recombination-deficient mutant cells of *Bacillus subtilis. Cancer Res.*, **36**, 445–451 (1976).

22. Ueno, Y., Kubota, K., Ito, T., and Nakamura, U. Mutagenicity of carcinogenic mycotoxins in *Salmonella typhimurium. Cancer Res.*, **38**, 538–542 (1978).

23. Ueno, Y., Yoshizawa, H., Uchimaru, R., Ito, T., and Tashiro, F. Nuclear envelope-dependent binding of aflatoxin B_1 to DNA. *In* "IUPAC Symposium on Mycotoxins and Phycotoxins," ed. P. Krogh, in press. Pathotox, Park Forest South, Ill.

24. Ueno, Y., Ishii, K., Omata, Y., Kamataki, T., and Kato, R. Specificity of hepatic cytochrome P-450 isoenzymes from PCB-treated rats and participation of cytochrome b_5 in the activation of aflatoxin B_1. *Carcinogenesis*, **4**, 1071–1073 (1983).

25. Vaught, J. B., Klohs, W., and Gurtoo, H. L. *In vitro* metabolism of aflatoxin B_1 by rat liver nuclei. *Life Sci.*, **21**, 1497–1504 (1977).

26. Wong, J. J. and Hsieh, D.P.H. Mutagenicity of aflatoxins related to their metabolism and carcinogenic potential. *Proc. Natl. Acad. Sci. U. S.*, **73**, 2241–2244 (1976).

27. Yoshizawa, H., Uchimaru, R., and Ueno, Y. Metabolism of aflatoxin B_1 in the nuclei isolated from rat liver. *J. Biochem.*, **89**, 443–452 (1981).

28. Yoshizawa, H., Uchimaru, R., Kamataki, T., Kato, R., and Ueno, Y. Metabolism and activation of aflatoxin B_1 by reconstituted cytochrome P-450 system of rat liver. *Cancer Res.*, **42**, 1120–1124 (1982).

GANN Monograph on Cancer Research 30, 1985

METABOLIC ACTIVATION OF 7,12-DIMETHYLBENZ[a]-ANTHRACENE AND 7-METHYLBENZ[a]ANTHRACENE *VIA* HYDROXYMETHYL SULFATE ESTERS BY P-450-SULFOTRANSFERASE

Tadashi WATABE,[*1] Tsuneo ISHIZUKA,[*1] Toshiko AIZAWA,[*1]
Yoshiki HAKAMATA,[*1] Akira HIRATSUKA,[*1] Kenichiro OGURA,[*1] and
Masakazu ISOBE[*2]

*Laboratory of Drug Metabolism and Toxicology, Department of Hygienic
Chemistry, Tokyo College of Pharmacy[*1] and Faculty of
Pharmaceutical Sciences, University of Setsunan[*2]*

7-Hydroxymethyl-12-methylbenz[a]anthracene (7-HMBA) and 12-hydroxymethyl-7-methylbenz[a]anthracene (12-HMBA), both carcinogenic major metabolites of 7,12-dimethylbenz[a]anthracene by cytochrome P-450 in untreated rat liver microsomes, yielded their sulfate ester conjugates as highly reactive and intrinsically mutagenic metabolites by the catalytic action of hepatic cytosolic sulfotransferase. 7-HMBA sulfate was enzymatically inactivated with glutathione (GSH) by GSH S-transferase in liver and non-enzymatically bound to hepatic cytosolic proteins and calf thymus DNA added through its 7-methylene group with loss of sulfate anion as a leaving group. S-cysteinyl, S-methionyl, and ε-N-lysyl adducts were isolated from the carcinogen-bound proteins, and N^6-adenyl and N^2-guanyl adducts from the DNA. These adducts as well as the conjugates were all identified with the corresponding synthetic specimens. 7-Hydroxymethylbenz[a]anthracene, a carcinogenic major metabolite of 7-methylbenz[a]anthracene by rat liver P-450, also yielded highly mutagenic 7-HBA sulfate by hepatic cytosolic sulfotransferase, which covalently bound to DNA and proteins.

Attention has long been paid to the question of why the carcinogenic activity of why the carcinogenic activity of benz[a]anthracene (BA), a very weak carcinogen, increases to the level of the most potent carcinogenic hydrocarbons, such as benzo[a]-pyrene (BP) and 3-methylcholanthrene (MC), with the substitution of methyl group(s) for the "L-region" (7- and 12-positions) hydrogens. For instance 7,12-dimethyl-BA (DMBA) has a higher carcinogenic activity than BP, and 7-methyl-BA (7-MBA) is as carcinogenic as MC (*6, 16*). In addition, MC is also an alkyl-substituted BA. The marked increase in carcinogenicity of aromatic hydrocarbons by a methyl substituent is observed not only with BA but also with other aromatic hydrocarbons such as chrysene and anthracene (*6, 16*). 5-Methylchrysene, for instance, has as highly carcinogenic

---

[*1] Horinouchi 1432-1, Hachioji, Tokyo 192-03, Japan (渡部　烈, 石塚恒雄, 会澤淑子, 袴田芳樹, 平塚明, 小倉健一郎).

[*2] Nagaotoge-cho 45-1, Hirakata, Osaka 537-01, Japan (磯部正和).

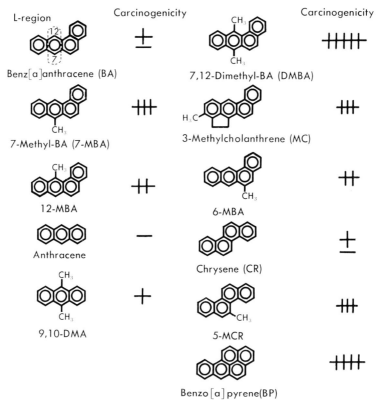

Fig. 1.   Increase in carcinogenicity of polycyclic hydrocarbons by methylation (from Cavalieri *et al.* (*6*); Selkirk (*16*)).

activity as MC, whereas the carcinogenicity of chrysene is very weak. Similarly, 9,10-dimethylanthracene is carcinogenic whereas the mother compound, anthracene, is not (Fig. 1).

Several attempts have been made to determine active metabolites of DMBA in relation to epoxide formation. DMBA 5,6-oxide has been isolated and identified as an active metabolite from a hepatic microsomal reaction mixture (*12*). DMBA 3,4-diol-1,2-epoxide was also assumed to be an active metabolite, but has not been yet detected in the *in vitro* system (*10, 14, 22*). These studies, however, were carried out using liver microsomes from rats pretreated with the P-448 inducer, MC or polychlorinated biphenyls. 8,9- and 10,11-epoxides of DMBA might also be candidates for the active metabolites since their hydrolysis products, 8,9- and 10,11-dihydrodiols, have been isolated from the rat liver microsomal system (*7*). It is of interest that 1,2,3,4-tetrahydro-DMBA still has carcinogenicity to mice skin (*8, 13*). This would suggest that DMBA is not necessarily activated *via* the bay region diol-epoxide.

Hydroxymethyl Sulfate Esters as Active Metabolites of Arylmethanols

Oxidation of DMBA occurs predominantly at the 7- and 12-carbons rather than aromatic carbons in untreated rat liver (*3*). The oxidation products, 7-hydroxymethyl-

12-methyl-BA (7-HMBA) and 12-hydroxymethyl-7-methyl-BA (12-HMBA), have been demonstrated to be potent carcinogens (4). The present study was undertaken to learn the metabolic activation mechanisms which involve HMBAs as proximate forms. *Salmonella typhimurium* TA strain bacteria (1) were used for detecting active metabolites.

7- and 12-HMBAs showed weak mutagenic activities toward *S. typhimurium* TA 98 in the presence of an untreated rat liver $9,000 \times g$ supernatnat fraction (S-9) fortified with an NADPH-generating system. However, their bacterial mutagenicity was markedly enhanced by the addition of ATP and sodium sulfate, a 3'-phosphoadenosine 5'-phosphosulfate (PAPS)-generating system, to the S-9 mixture (Table I).

TABLE I. Mutagenicity of 7-HMBA, 12-HMBA, and DMBA toward *S. typhimurium* TA98 in the Presence of an Untreated Rat Liver $9,000 \times g$ Supernatant Fraction (S-9)

Carcinogen	Preincubation system[a]	No. of His+ revertant colonies/plate
None	S-9+NADPH	24
	S-9+PAPS	23
	S-9+NADPH+PAPS	23
7-HMBA[b]	S-9+NADPH	83
	S-9+PAPS	863
12-HMBA[b]	S-9+NADPH	179
	S-9+PAPS	746
DMBA	S-9+NADPH	474
	S-9+NADPH+PAPS	636
BP	S-9+NADPH	683

[a] The preincubation system consisted of the following in a final volume of 1 ml of 0.1 M Na_2HPO_4-KH_2PO_4 buffer, pH 7.4: bacterial cells (10^9), dimethyl sulfoxide (0.1 ml) dissolving the carcinogen (1 mM), S-9 (8 mg of protein, equivalent to 50 mg of liver, wet weight), $MgCl_2$ (3 mM), EDTA (0.1 mM), PAPS generated from Na_2SO_4 (5 mM), and ATP (5 mM), or/and NADPH generated from NADP (4 mM) and glucose 6-phosphate (5 mM). S-9 was reconstituted of washed microsomes and dialyzed S-105 ($105,000 \times g$ supernatant fraction). Preincubations were carried out for 20 min at 37° before dilution with soft agar.
[b] S-9 used was reconstituted of microsomes and S-105 from 50 and 30 mg of liver, respectively. A significant decrease in number of His+ revertant colonies, due to the cytotoxic effect of HMBAs, occurred at higher amounts of S-105.

TABLE II. Mutagenicity of 7-HMBA and 12-HMBA toward *S. typhimurium* TA98 in the Presence of Untreated Rat Liver Cytosol (S-105) and PAPS-generating System

Preincubation system	No. of His+ revertant colonies/plate	
	7-HMBA	12-HMBA
Complete[a]	988	856
-HMBA	39	39
-S-105	39	42
-ATP	42	38
-Na_2SO_4	41	45
Complete (boiled S-105)[a]	40	41

[a] The complete preincubation system consisted of S-105 (equivalent to 30 mg liver) and the same ingredients except NADP and glucose 6-phosphate as those described in Table I.

DMBA also showed a higher mutagenicity in the presence of both NADPH- and PAPS-generating systems than in the presence of the NADPH-generating system alone. Under the same conditions, the maximum bacterial mutagenicity of BP in the presence of the NADPH-generating system was lower than that of 7- or 12-HMBA in the presence of the PAPS-generating system.

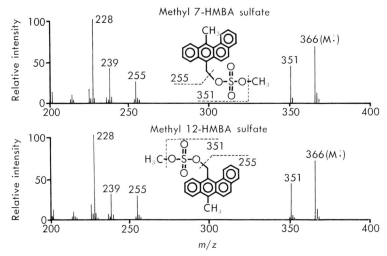

FIG. 2.   GLC-MS of methyl esters of metabolically formed 7- and 12-HMBA sulfates. GLC conditions: a 1% OV-1 column (60–80 mesh Chromosorb W, 3 mm × 1 m) eluted with 40 ml helium/min at 290°. Retention times of the methyl esters were 4.5 and 6.1 min for 7- and 12-HMBA sulfates, respectively.

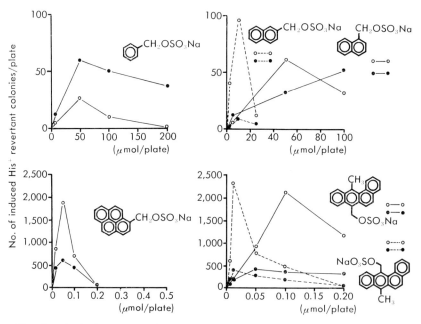

FIG. 3.   Intrinsic mutagenicity of arylmethyl sulfates toward *S. typhimurium* TA 98 and TA 100. ○ TA 98; ● TA 100.

S-9 could be replaced by a dialyzed soluble supernatant fraction (S-105) to activate 7- and 12-HMBAs. Similar to the case of S-9, their mutagenic activities were reduced to the background level either when S-105 was boiled or when ATP or sodium sulfate was omitted from the incubation mixture (Table II).

From a mixture consisting of 7- or 12-HMBA, S-105, and the PAPS-generating system, a water-soluble, directly acting mutagen was isolated by an Amberlite XAD-2 column adsorption method. The polar mutagens from 7- and 12-HMBAs were identified by UV absorption spectroscopy, thin layer chromatography (TLC) and high pressure liquid chromatography (HPLC) with their sulfate esters. These were synthesized from the promutagenic alcohols by the reaction with freshly redistilled chlorosulfonic acid in dry pyridine, followed by careful neutralization with a diluted methanolic sodium hydroxide solution. The biologically formed active metabolites were also identified as 7- and 12-HMBA sulfuric acid esters by gas-liquid chromatography-mass spectroscopy (GLC-MS) after derivatization of the free acids with diazomethane (Fig. 2) (19).

Synthetic sodium sulfate esters of arylmethanols, benzyl alcohol, 1- and 2-naphthyl-methanols, 1-pyrenylmethanol, 7- and 12-HMBAs all showed mutagenic activity toward *S. typhimurium* TA 98 and TA 100 strain bacteria. Only benzyl sulfate showed a higher mutagenicity toward TA 100 than toward TA 98, and the others *vice versa*. Their mutagenicity increased with the increase in number of aromatic rings (19) (Fig. 3). Mutagenicity of 7-hydroxymethyl-BA sulfate ester toward *Salmonella* has also been reported by Cavalieri *et al.* (6). However, sulfate esters of methanol, ethanol, *n*-propanol, and *n*-butanol showed no intrinsic mutagenicity toward either strain of bacteria.

Inactivation of 7-HMBA Sulfate by GSH S-Transferase

The bacterial mutagenicity of 7-HMBA was markedly retarded by the addition of glutathione (GSH) to the incubation mixture consisting of S-105 and the PAPS-generating system. From the incubation mixture without the bacteria was isolated a non-mutagenic, ninhydrin-positive conjugate identified as S-(12-methyl-BA-7-ly) methylglutathione (GSH) with the corresponding synthetic specimen by TLC, HPLC, and UV absorption spectroscopy (20). The same GSH conjugate was yielded at a much higher rate from 7-HMBA sulfate by S-105. The conjugation reaction of the sulfate also proceeded at a very slow rate in the absence of S-105. However, with enhancement of the pH of the non-enzymatic reaction medium up to 9.0, the rate was remarkably accelerated with concomitant formation of an increasing amount of 7-HMBA. The GSH conjugate afforded S-(12-methyl-BA-7-yl)methylcysteine, glutamic acid, and glycine on heating at 100° in 10N HCl and nitrogen as a gaseous phase. The S-cysteinyl derivative was identified with the product obtained by the reaction of 7-HMBA sulfate and L-cysteine at pH 9.0 and room temperature. Thus, it is evident that 7-HMBA is activated by sulfotransferase to its sulfate ester and inactivated by GSH S-transferase to the GSH conjugate in rat liver cytosol.

Covalent Binding of 7-HMBA Sulfate to Hepatic Cytosolic Proteins

7-HMBA existed in a protein-bound form rather than in a free one in the incuba-tion mixture consisting of S-105 and the PAPS-generating system. Hepatic soluble protein precipitated from the mixture by the addition of trichloroacetic acid was thoroughly washed and hydrolyzed at 100° for 1 hr with 10N HCl in nitrogen as a gaseous phase. The acid hydrolyzate showed an intense fluorescence spectrum characteristic of a DMBA chromophor after exhaustive extraction with ether. The fluorescence was completely adsorbed on an Amberlite XAD-2 column and eluted from it with methanol. The methanolic eluate showed a cluster of peaks due to very polar materials and two well-isolated single peaks at longer retention times on an octadecylsilicone (ODS) column by monitoring at 293 nm (Fig. 4). A UV-absorbing peak showing the DMBA chromophor moved from the cluster peaks into a longer retention time region when they were eluted and re-chromatographed in aqueous methanol containing triethylamine as a counter ion. The three peak materials having the DMBA chromophor which were isolated from the chromatograms showed single spots visualized by ninhydrin and a UV lamp for fluorescence emission (Fig. 4).

The two less polar amino acid adducts were identified not only by UV spectroscopy but also by MS after trifluoroacetyl-methylation with trifluoroacetic anhydride and diazomethane in the standard manner as ε-N-(12-methyl-BA-7-ly)methyllysine and S-(12-methyl-BA-7-ly)methylcysteine with authentic specimens synthesized from 7-HMBA sulfate and L-lysine and L-cysteine at pH 9.0, respectively. The latter adduct was identical with that obtained from the GSH conjugate of 7-HMBA sulfate by acid hydrolysis. The most polar amino acid adduct was identified by HPLC, TLC, and UV absorption spectroscopy as S-(12-methyl-BA-7-ly)methylmethionine with an authentic specimen synthesized from 7-HMBA sulfate and L-methionine at pH 9.0. Furthermore, it was derivatized to a less polar, ninhydrin-positive adduct, which was less polar than the cysteine adduct, by heating with methanolic sodium hydroxide in nitrogen. The

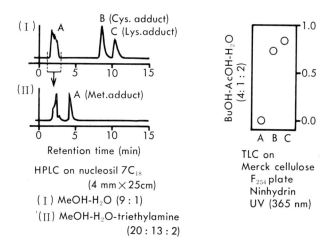

FIG. 4. Chromatographic separation and identification of carcinogen-amino acid adducts from an acid hydrolyzate of hepatic cytosolic proteins treated with 7-HMBA in the presence of a PAPS-generating system or with 7-HMBA sulfate in the absence of the cofactor system. A in HPL-chromatogram (I) was eluted and re-chromatographed under the illustrated conditions (II). The chromatograms were monitored at 293 nm (left). The adducts separated by HPLC were also re-chromatographed by TLC (right).

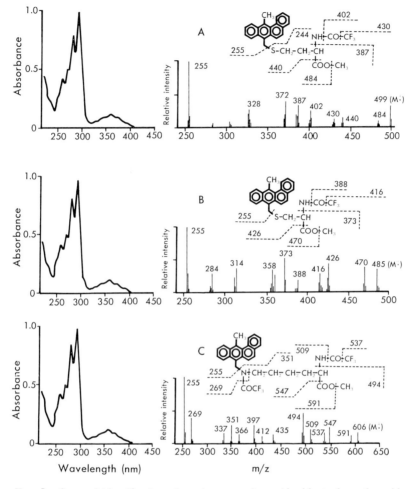

FIG. 5. Spectral identification of carcinogen-amino acid adducts from the acid hydrolyzate of hepatic cytosolic proteins treated with 7-HMBA in the presence of the PAPS-generating system or with 7-HMBA sulfate alone (Watabe et al. (21)). The amino acid adducts were isolated by HPLC as illustrated in Fig. 4. Ultraviolet absorption spectra of the adducts were recorded in methanol before trifluoroacetyl-methylation. The homocysteine adduct (A) was derivatized from the methionine adduct. Cysteine (B) and lysine (C) adducts.

less polar product was also characterized by MS as S-(12-methyl-BA-7-ly)methylhomocysteine after the derivatization (Fig. 5). The cysteinyl SH of the hepatic protein was the most susceptible to the adduct formation with 7-HMBA sulfate, and the methionyl S was next (21).

Covalent Binding of 7-HMBA Sulfate to DNA

7-HMBA covalently bound to calf thymus DNA 4 times more than to S-105 protein when incubated in the presence of the PAPS-generating system. That is, the binding ratio of 7-HMBA (0.1 mM) to DNA (1 mg/ml) was 1.4 nmol/mg DNA and to

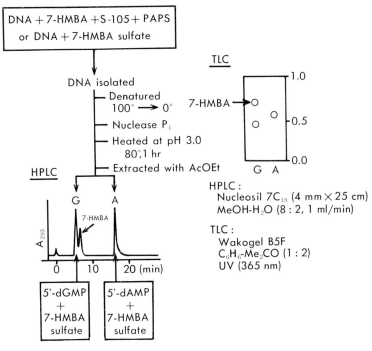

FIG. 6. Chromatographic separation and identification of carcinogen-DNA base adducts. The reaction mixtures of the 5'-mononucleotides with 7-HMBA sulfate were heated at pH 3.0 and 80° and then extracted with ethyl acetate. TLC was carried out with the HPLC peak materials eluted from the column.

S-105 proteins 1.25 nmol/mg protein when incubated for 20 min with S-105 (3.5 mg protein/ml) in the presence of the PAPS-generating system. DNA that was isolated in a protein-free form from the mixture and thoroughly washed with organic solvents showed an intense fluorescence spectrum characteristic of the DMBA chromophor. The spectrum, however, was not detectable when S-105 was boiled or when either ATP or sodium sulfate was omitted from the mixture. The fluorescence substance was not eliminated by extraction with ethyl acetate from the isolated DNA after it was denatured by heating followed by rapid cooling and well digested by nuclease P_1. However, 76% of the fluorescence emitted from the enzymatic digest was extracted into ethyl acetate after it was heated at 80° and pH 3.0 for 1 hr. The ethyl acetate layer was found by ODS-HPLC and silica-TLC to contain three UV-absorbing or fluorescence materials (Fig. 6), one of which was identified with 7-HMBA by UV absorption spectroscopy and MS, and the others were suggested by MS to be adducts of 7-HMBA to guanine and adenine with loss of a water molecule (Fig. 7). The same chromatographic and mass spectroscopic results were obtained after incubation of calf thymus DNA with 7-HMBA sulfate at pH 7.4 in the absence of S-105 and the PAPS-generating system, followed by the treatments with nuclease P_1 and at pH 3.0. However, covalent binding of the sulfate to DNA occurred at a much higher rate than that by the metabolic activation system. A fluorophotometric study indicated that a maximum binding ratio of 7-HMBA sulfate (0.1 mM) to DNA (1 mg/ml) reached 1 to 30 bp.

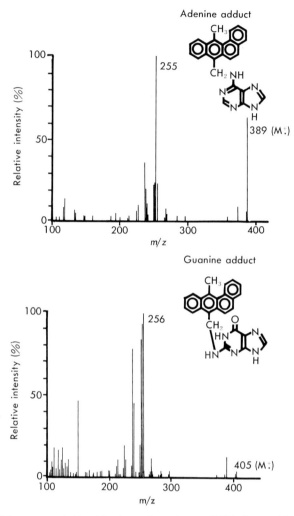

FIG. 7. Mass spectral identification of carcinogen-DNA base adducts. Mass spectra were recorded with materials corresponding to peaks A and G eluted from the HPL-chromatogram in Fig. 6.

The purely isolated guanine adduct was found to be labile at pH 3.0 and 80° and to yield 7-HMBA slowly with concomitant loss of the adduct, whereas the adenine adduct was quite stable under these conditions. The HPL-chromatogram in Fig. 6 indicated that the guanine and adenine adducts existed in the molar ratio 3:2 in the DNA so far as estimated from the three peak areas. The adenine and guanine adducts from DNA, treated with 7-HMBA in the presence of the hepatic sulfotransferase system or directly with 7-HMBA sulfate, were identical in all respects with the products obtained by the reactions of 7-HMBA sulfate at pH 9.0 with 5′-dAMP and 5′-dGMP, respectively, followed by heating at pH 3.0 (Fig. 6). The reactions of 7-HMBA sulfate with the 5′-mononucleotides also proceeded at pH 7.4 and yielded the same adducts, but the rates were much slower than those at pH 9.0. The reaction of the sulfate with

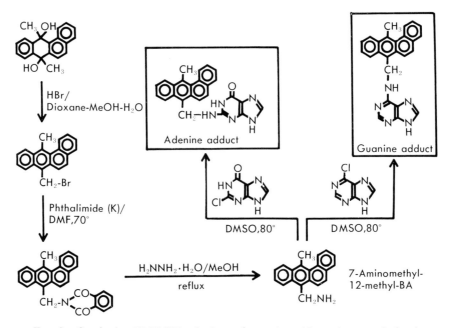

Fig. 8.   Synthesis of 7-HMBA-adenine and -guanine adducts that were isolated
from DNA treated with 7-HMBA sulfate or with 7-HMBA in the presence of
rat liver cytosol fortified with a PAPS-generating system. 7-Aminomethyl-12-
methyl-BA (NMR $\delta_{\mathrm{TMS}}^{\mathrm{CDCl_3}}$ ppm: 3.35 (s, 3H, 12-CH$_3$), 4.77 (broad s, 2H, 7-CH$_2$-),
7.33–8.13 (m, 10H, arom. H); IR $\nu_{\max}^{\mathrm{KBr}}$ cm^{-1} (as HCl salt): 2,900 (broad), 1,560,
1,490, 1,360, 1,120; UV $\lambda_{\max}^{\mathrm{EtOH}}$ nm (ε): 213 (16,520), 235 (10,375), 263 (17,750),
273 (20,910), 283 (31,500), 294 (32,710), 328 (2,431), 342 (3,992), 360 (5,345), 377
(4,170)) was synthesized from the 7,12-dimethyl-7,12-diol in almost quantitative
yield without pruification and reacted at a concentration of 40 mM for 1 hr with
1.3 molar ratio of 2-chloro-6-hydroxy- and 6-chloro-purines in nitrogen as a
gaseous phase. The products were isolated by silica gel chromatography and
recrystallized from acetic acid-methanol for the guanine adduct and from acetone-
methanol for the adenine adduct.

DNA at pH 7.4, however, proceeded much faster than those with the mono-nucleotides
at pH 9.0.

A synthetic approach was made to determine the positions of the nucleic acid bases
to which the carcinogen was attached through its 7-methylene group. Reactions of the
key compound, 7-aminomethyl-12-methyl-BA, with commercially available 6-chloro-
purine and 2-chloro-6-hydroxy-purine afforded the adenine and guanine adducts in
80 and 50% yields, respectively, which were identical with the adducts from DNA
by HPLC, TLC, MS, UV absorption spectroscopy, and fluorospectroscopy (Fig. 8).
The synthetic guanine adduct slowly decomposed at pH 3.0 and 80° with concomitant
formation of 7-HMBA, whereas the synthetic adenine adduct was resistant to acid
hydrolysis.

Thus, a novel metabolic activation mechanism for DMBA has been established
as illustrated in Fig. 9, focusing only the role of the 7-methyl group. The mechanism
involves oxidation at the L-region methyl group by microsomal P-450 to yield 7-HMBA
and sulfuric acid conjugation by cytosolic sulfotransferase to yield reactive 7-HMBA

sulfate as an ultimate form. The sulfate moiety of the conjugate acts as a leaving group, so that the benzylic carbon may be readily attacked by nucleophilic functional groups

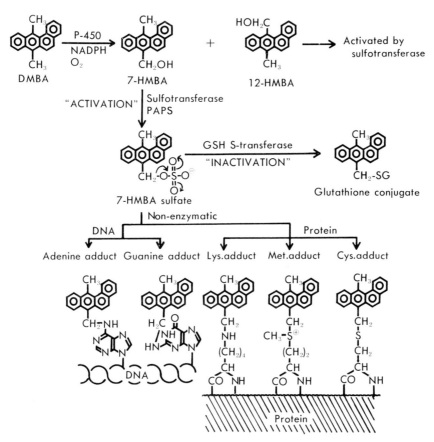

FIG. 9.   Metabolic activation, inactivation, and covalent binding to biomacromolecules of 7-HMBA, a proximate carcinogen of DMBA.

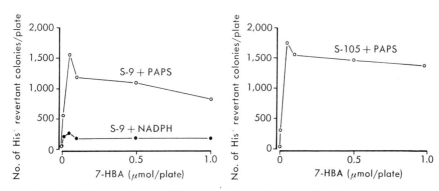

FIG. 10.   Mutagenicity of 7-HBA toward *S. typhimurium* TA 98 in the presence of an untreated rat liver S-9 or S-105. S-9 used was reconstituted of washed microsomes and dialyzed S-105 both equivalent to 50 mg of rat liver. PAPS and NADPH were generated from the corresponding cofactor-generating systems. Mutagenicity tests were carried out under the same conditions as described in Table I.

of biomacromolecules and GSH. The observed higher rate in covalent binding of 7-HMBA sulfate to DNA than to hepatic cytosolic proteins may suggest that the rate-limiting step for the binding would be an intercalation of the water-soluble, active metabolite to the DNA molecule through its arene moiety.

7-HBA Sulfate as an Active Metabolite of 7-MBA

7-MBA also showed a much higher mutagenicity toward *S. typhimurium* TA 98 by untreated rat liver S-9 in the presence of the NADPH- and PAPS-generating systems than in the presence of the NADPH-generating system alone. 7-HBA, a major metabolite of 7-MBA in rat liver (*17, 18*) and a potent carcinogen (*5*), was potently activated

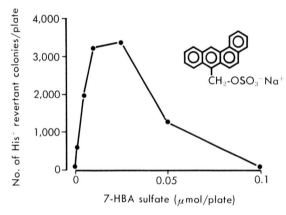

FIG. 11. Intrinsic mutagenicity of 7-HBA sulfate toward *S. typhimurium* TA 98. The mutagenicity test was carried out under the same conditions as described in Fig. 3.

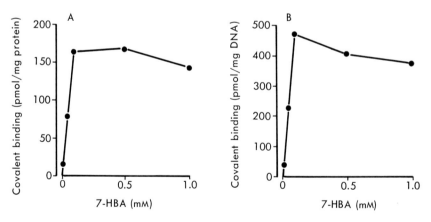

FIG. 12. Covalent binding of 7-HBA toward biomacromolecules in the presence of an untreated rat liver cytosol and a PAPS-generating system. A: the incubation mixture consisted of rat liver S-105 (from 500 mg liver), 7-HBA (in 1 ml DMSO), ATP (5 mM), Na₂SO₄ (5 mM), MgCl₂ (3 mM), and EDTA (0.1 mM) in a final volume of 10 ml of 0.1 M phosphate buffer, pH 7.4. B: to the above incubation mixture was added calf thymus DNA (20 mg).

by either S-9 or S-105 in the presence of the PAPS-generating system, but was less activated by the S-9-NADPH system (Fig. 10) than was 7-MBA.

From the incubation mixture was isolated the reactive metabolite, 7-HBA sulfate on an Amberlite XAD-2 column, which was identified by UV absorption spectroscopy with the corresponding synthetic specimen after being separated by ODS-HPLC. Both metabolically formed and synthetic 7-HBA sulfates had intrinsic mutagenicity toward *S. typhimurium* TA 98 (Fig. 11) and covalently bound to DNA as well as to S-105 proteins at lower ratios than 7- and 12-HMBA sulfates (Figs. 12 and 13). DNA was more susceptible to covalent binding by both metabolically formed and synthetic 7-HBA sulfates than S-105 proteins.

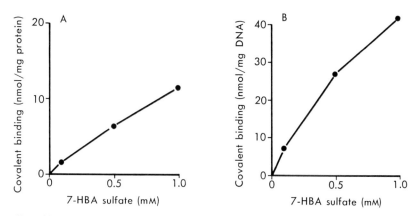

Fig. 13.   Covalent binding of 7-HBA sulfate toward biomacromolecules. A: the incubation mixture consisted of S-105 (from 50 mg liver) of a male Wistar rat liver homogenate and 7-HBA sulfate (in 0.1 ml DMSO) in a final volume of 1 ml of 0.1 M phosphate buffer, pH 7.4. B: the incubation mixture consisted of calf thymus DNA (2 mg) and 7-HBA sulfate (in 0.1 ml DMSO) in a final volume of 1 ml of 0.1 M phosphate buffer, pH 7.4.

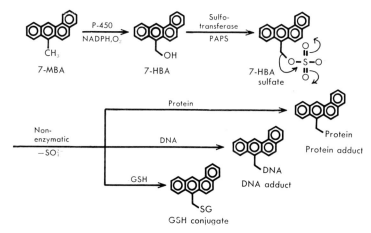

Fig. 14.   Metabolic activation, inactivation and covalent binding to biomacromolecules of 7-HBA, a proximate carcinogen of 7-MBA.

7-HBA sulfate had a much shorter half life than 7-HMBA sulfate at pH 7.4 and 37° and was non-enzymatically scavenged by GSH to yield non-mutagenic S-(BA-7-yl)methylglutathione. These results are illustrated in Fig. 14.

7-HMBA phosphate has been assumed to be a reactive intermediate non-enzymatically formed from 7-HMBA and ATP alone as well as from ATP, sodium sulfate and rat liver cytosol (9). However, the possibility of the participation of the putative phosphoric acid ester was completely excluded by the present investigation.

The possibility has been proposed by Miller and his co-workers of the participation of hepatic sulfotransferase in the metabolic activation of N-OH-FAA, N-OH-MAB, and 1'-hydroxysafrole (2, 11, 15). However, they failed to obtain direct evidence for the formation of reactive sulfuric acid conjugates with these carcinogens. Evidence for the directly acting carcinogen of a sulfate ester of an aralkyl alcohol has been provided with 6-hydroxymethyl-BP (6). However, it is still equivocal whether or not the sulfate is biologically formed.

Therefore, the present investigation provides the first direct evidence of biological formation of the reactive sulfuric acid esters of carcinogens and their binding to bio-macromolecules.

REFERENCES

1. Ames, B. N., McCann, J., and Yamasaki, E. Methods of detecting carcinogens and mutagens with the *Salmonella*/mammalian-microsome mutagenicity test. *Mut. Res.*, **31**, 347–363 (1975).

2. Boberg, E. W., Miller, E. C., Miller, J. R., Poland, A., and Liem, A. Strong evidence from studies with brachymorphic mice and pentachlorophenol that 1'-sulfoöxysafrole is the major ultimate electrophilic and carcinogenic metabolite of 1'-hydroxysafrole in mouse liver. *Cancer Res.*, **43**, 5163–5173 (1983).

3. Boyland, E. and Sims, P. Metabolism of polycyclic compounds: the metabolism of 7,12-dimethylbenz[a]anthracene by rat-liver homogenates. *Biochem. J.*, **95**, 780–787 (1965).

4. Boyland, E. and Sims, P. The carcinogenic activities in mice of compounds related to benz[a]anthracene. *Int. J. Cancer*, **2**, 500–504 (1967).

5. Cavalieri, E., Roth, R., Rogan, E., Grandjean, C., and Althoff, J. Mechanisms of tumor initiation. *In* "Carcinogenesis", ed. P. W. Jones and R. I. Freudenthal, pp. 273–284 (1978). Raven Press, New York.

6. Cavalieri, E., Roth, R., and Rogan, E. Hydroxylation and conjugation at the benzylic carbon atom: A possible mechanism of carcinogenic activation for some methyl-substituted aromatic hydrocarbons. *In* "Polynuclear Aromatic Hydrocarbons," ed. P. W. Jones and P. Leber, pp. 517–529 (1979). Ann Arbor Science Publishers, Ann Arbor, Michigan.

7. DiGiovanni, J. and Juchau, M. R. Biotransformation and bioactivation of 7,12-dimethylbenz[a]anthracene (7,12-DMBA). *Drug Metab. Rev.*, **11**, 61–101 (1980).

8. DiGiovanni, J., Diamond, L., Singer, J. M., Daniel, F. B., Witiak, D. T., and Slaga, T. J. Tumor-initiating activity of 4-fluoro-7, 12-dimethylbenz[a]anthracene and 1, 2, 3, 4-tetrahydro-7, 12-dimethylbenz[a]anthracene in female SENCAR mice. *Carcinogenesis*, **3**, 651–655 (1982).

9. Flesher, J. W. and Tay, L. K. Reactions of the carcinogens 7-hydroxymethyl-12-methylbenz[a]anthracene and 7-acetoxymethyl-12-methylbenz[a]anthracene with DNA. *Res. Commun. Chem. Pathol. Pharmacol.*, **22**, 345–355 (1978).

10. Jerina, D. M., Yagi, H., Lehr, R. E., Thakker, D. R., Schaefer-Ridder, M., Karle, J. M., Levin, W., Wood, A. W., Chang, R. L., and Conney, A. H. The bay region theory of carcinogenesis by polycyclic aromatic hydrocarbons. *In* "Polycyclic Hydrocarbons and Cancer," ed. H. V. Gelboin and P. O. P. Ts'o, Vol. 1, pp. 173–188 (1978). Academic Press, New York.

11. Kadlubar, F. F., Miller, J. A., and Miller, E. C. Hepatic metabolism of *N*-hydroxy-*N*-methyl-4-aminoazobenzene and other *N*-hydroxyarylamines to reactive sulfuric acid esters. *Cancer Res.*, **36**, 2350–2359 (1976).

12. Keysell, G. R., Booth, J., Grover, P. L., Hewer, A., and Sims, P. The formation of "K-region" epoxides as hepatic microsomal metabolites of 7-methylbenz[a]anthracene and 7,12-dimethylbenz[a]anthracene and their 7-hydroxymethyl derivatives. *Biochem. Pharmacol.*, **22**, 2853–2867 (1973).

13. Lijinsky, W., Manning, W. B., and Andrews, A. W. Skin carcinogenesis tests in mice of derivatives of 7,12-dimethylbenz[a]anthracene substituted in the 'A' ring. *Carcinogenesis*, **4**, 1221–1224 (1983).

14. Malaveille, C., Bartsch, H., Tierney, B., Grover, P. L., and Sims, P. Microsome-mediated mutagenicities of dihydrodiols of 7,12-dimethylbenz[a]anthracene: High mutagenic activity of the 3,4-dihydrodiol. *Biochem. Biophys. Res. Commun.*, **83**, 1468–1473 (1978).

15. Miller, J. A. and Miller, E. C. The concept of reactive electrophilic metabolites in chemical carcinogenesis: Recent results with aromatic amines, safrole, and aflatoxin B$_1$. *In* "Biological Reactive Intermediates," ed. D. J. Jollow, J. J. Kocsis, R. Snyder, and H. Vainio, pp. 6–24 (1977). Plenum Press, New York and London.

16. Selkirk, J. K. Chemical carcinogenesis: A brief overview of the mechanism of action of polycyclic hydrocarbons, aromatic amines, nitrosoamines, and aflatoxins. *In* "Carcinogenesis," ed. T. J. Slaga, Vol. 5, pp. 1–31 (1980). Raven Press, New York.

17. Sims, P. The metabolism of 7- and 12-methylbenz[a]anthracene and their derivatives. *Biochem. J.*, **105**, 591–598 (1967).

18. Sims, P. Qualitative and quantitative studies on the metabolism of a series of aromatic hydrocarbons by rat-liver preparations. *Biochem. Pharmacol.*, **19**, 795–818 (1970).

19. Watabe T., Ishizuka, T., Isobe, M., and Ozawa, N. A 7-hydroxymethyl sulfate ester as an active metabolite of 7,12-dimethylbenz[a]anthracene. *Science*, **215**, 403–405 (1982).

20. Watabe, T., Ishizuka, T., Ozawa, N., and Isobe, M. Conjugation of 7-hydroxymethyl-12-methylbenz[a]anthracene (7-HMBA) with glutathione *via* a sulfate ester in hepatic cytosol. *Biochem. Pharmacol.*, **31**, 2542–2544 (1982).

21. Watabe, T., Ishizuka, T., Hakamata, Y., Aizawa, T., and Isobe, M. Covalent binding of the proximate carcinogen, 7-hydroxymethyl-12-methylbenz[a]anthracene (7-HMBA), to the rat liver cytosolic protein *via* 7-HMBA sulfate. *Biochem. Pharmacol.*, **32**, 2120–2122 (1983).

22. Wislocki, P. G., Gadek, K. M., Chou, M. W., Yang, S. K., and Lu, A. Y. H. Carcinogenicity and mutagenicity of the 3,4-dihydrodiols and other metabolites of 7,12-dimethylbenz[a]anthracene and its hydroxymethyl derivatives. *Cancer Res.*, **40**, 3661–3664 (1980).

INDUCTION AND GENETICS
OF CYTOCHROME P-450

GANN Monograph on Cancer Research 30, 1985

INDUCTION OF MICROSOMAL CYTOCHROME P-450 IN RAT LIVER BY CHEMICAL COMPOUNDS

Tsuneo OMURA

Department of Biology, Faculty of Science, Kyushu University*

Two forms of cytochrome P-450, P-450(PB-1) and P-450(MC-1), were purified from the liver microsomes of phenobarbital(PB)-treated and 3-methylcholanthrene(MC)-treated rats, respectively, and their selective induction by PB or MC was confirmed using specific antibodies. 1,1-Di(*p*-chlorophenyl)-2,2-dichloroethylene (DDE), whose chemical structure is significantly different from that of PB, was also found to cause a highly selective induction of P-450(PB-1) in the liver microsomes of the treated animals.

Increased synthesis of P-450(PB-1) and P-450(MC-1) was mainly responsible for the selective and remarkable increase of those inducible forms of cytochrome P-450 by the inducers. The turnover rate of P-450 (PB-1) was not significantly affected by PB administration. The stimulated synthesis of P-450(PB-1) induced by PB or DDE was explained by a rapid increase of its mRNA in the livers of the treated animals.

The administration of certain chemical compounds such as phenobarbital (PB) and 3-methylcholanthrene (MC), induces microsomal cytochrome P-450-dependent drug oxidation activity in the livers of the treated animals, and the induction of the oxidation activity is usually accompanied by significant alterations in its substrate specificity (*4*). Since liver microsomes contain multiple molecular species of cytochrome P-450 having different substrate specificities, the drug-induced changes in the substrate specificity of the microsomal oxidation activity should be correlated with the alterations in the isozyme compositions of the microsomal cytochrome P-450. In order to obtain a clear picture of the induction of microsomal drug-oxidation activity, which is responsible for the metabolic activation of a wide variety of chemical carcinogens, the induction of microsomal cytochrome P-450 should be examined for each molecular species of cytochrome P-450. Various drug-inducible forms of cytochrome P-450 have been purified from the liver microsomes of treated animals, and immunochemical quantitation of particular forms of the cytochrome in the microsomes has recently been carried out (*6, 11–13, 18, 21, 23–26, 32–34*).

We purified four forms of cytochrome P-450 from the liver microsomes of PB-treated and MC-treated rats to examine their induction by xenobiotic compounds (*16*). This paper summarizes a series of our recent studies (*13, 14, 16, 19, 29, 30, 39*) on the induction of two major drug-inducible forms of cytochrome P-450, P-450(PB-1) and P-450(MC-1), in rat liver microsomes. We confirmed highly selective induction of

---

* Hakozaki 6-10-1, Higashi-ku, Fukuoka 812, Japan (大村恒雄).

P-450(PB-1) or P-450(MC-1) by a few chemical compounds. The increase of these particular forms of cytochrome P-450 in the liver microsomes could be explained by selective stimulation of their synthesis, which was caused by a rapid increase of specific mRNA in the livers of the treated animals.

Selective Induction of Different Molecular Species of Microsomal Cytochrome P-450 in Rat Liver by Phenobarbital and 3-Methylcholanthrene

P-450(PB-1) and P-450(MC-1) are the major components of cytochrome P-450 in the liver microsomes of PB-treated and MC-treated rats, respectively. They were purified to homogeneity from the liver microsomes of drug-treated male Sprague-Dawley rats (*13, 16*). The rabbit antibodies prepared against each of these two forms of cytochrome P-450 did not show cross immunoreaction, and the contents of P-450 (PB-1) and P-450(MC-1) in rat liver microsomes could be separately determined by quantitative immunoprecipitation of each of the antigens from detergent-solubilized microsomes (*13*).

As shown in Fig. 1, the administration of PB to rats resulted in a rapid selective increase of P-450(PB-1) in the liver microsomes, whereas the content of P-450(MC-1) did not increase at all. The contents of P-450(PB-1) and P-450(MC-1) in the liver microsomes of untreated rats were both 5–10% of total cytochrome P-450, but the content of P-450(PB-1) in the liver microsomes of PB-treated animals increased to 55–60% of total cytochrome P-450 24 hr after drug administration. Similarly, MC administration elevated the content of P-450(MC-1) in the liver microsomes of the treated animals without affecting the content of P-450(PB-1) (Fig. 2).

Selective increase of inducer-specific forms of cytochrome P-450 by PB and MC was first described by Thomas *et al.* (*32*), and confirmed by many similar reports (*6,*

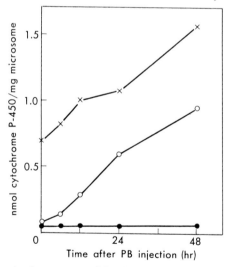

Fig. 1.   Changes in the contents of P-450(PB-1) and P-450(MC-1) in rat liver microsomes induced by PB administration to the animals (*13*). PB was injected intraperitoneally to a group of rats at time zero and 24 hr. Several rats were killed at each time point, and the contents of total cytochrome P-450 ($\times$), P-450(PB-1) (○), and P-450(MC-1) (●) in the liver microsomes were assayed.

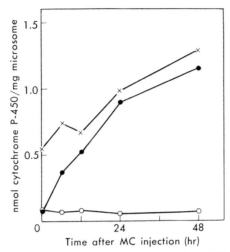

FIG. 2. Changes in the contents of P-450(PB-1) and P-450(MC-1) in rat liver microsomes induced by MC administration to the animals (*13*). MC was injected intraperitoneally to a group of rats at time zero, and the contents of total cytochrome P-450 ($\times$), P-450(PB-1) ($\bigcirc$), and P-450(MC-1) ($\bullet$) in the liver microsomes were assayed.

11, 12, 18, 21, 23–26, 33, 34), in which various immunochemical methods were utilized to quantitate particular forms of cytochrome P-450 in microsomes.

Induction of a Phenobarbital-inducible Form of Microsomal Cytochrome P-450 by 1,1-Di(p-chlorophenyl)-2,2-dichloroethylene

Although P-450(PB-1) and P-450(MC-1) were selectively induced by PB and MC, respectively, the number of inducible forms of cytochrome P-450 in liver microsomes seems to be rather limited. It is therefore unlikely that a large number of xenobiotic compounds, which have been found to induce cytochrome P-450 in liver microsomes, correspond with the same number of different forms of cytochrome P-450. The xenobiotic inducers can probably be grouped into several types, each of which corresponds mainly to one inducible form of cytochrome P-450.

Depending on the substrate specificity of the induced drug oxidation activity, xenobiotic inducers are usually divided into two types, PB-type inducers and MC-type inducers. The former are characterized by a strong stimulation of the oxidative N-demethylation of benzphetamine, aminopyrene, *etc.*, whereas the latter stimulate the ring hydroxylation activity to various aromatic hydrocarbons. We examined a PB-type inducer, 1,1-di(*p*-chlorophenyl)-2,2-dichloroethylene (DDE), and found that the compound, whose chemical structure is significantly different from that of PB, induced P-450(PB-1) in the liver microsomes of treated rats. DDE is a metabolite of 1,1-di(*p*-chlorophenyl)-2,2,2-trichloroethane (DDT), and is highly resistant to further metabolic degradation in animals (*15*).

When DDE was intraperitoneally injected to rats, it induced a persistent elevation of the drug oxidation activity of the liver microsomes, which remained at a high level until about 10 days after a single dose of DDE (*39*). When the content of cytochrome

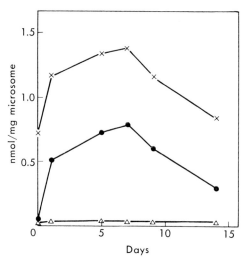

Fig. 3. Effect of DDE on the contents of P-450(PB-1) and P-450(MC-1) in rat liver microsomes (39). The contents of P-450(PB-1) and P-450(MC-1) in the liver microsomes from DDE-treated rats were measured by immunoprecipitation using specific antibodies. The contents of total cytochrome P-450 (×), P-450 (PB-1) (●), and P-450 (MC-1) (△) are shown in the figure.

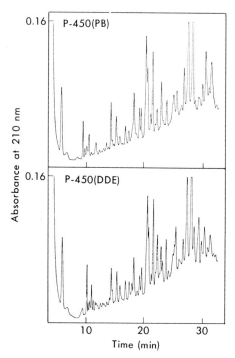

Fig. 4. Comparison of the tryptic peptides from P-450(DDE) and P-450(PB-1) by reverse phase HPLC (39). Each of P-450(DDE) and P-450(PB-1) was subjected to digestion with TPC-treated trypsin, and the peptides were separated by reverse phase HPLC.

P-450 in the liver microsomes was examined, it was found to increase almost in parallel with the increase of drug oxidation activity, and the immunochemical characterization of its molecular species in the microsomes indicated that the increase of total cytochrome P-450 was fully explained by an increase of a form of cytochrome P-450 which was immunochemically identical to P-450(PB-1) (Fig. 3). A major form of cytochrome P-450 was purified from the liver microsomes of DDE-treated rats, and the molecular and immunochemical properties of the purified cytochrome P-450, P-450(DDE), were found to be identical with those of P-450(PB-1) (39). Figure 4 shows the tryptic peptide maps of P-450(PB-1) and P-450(DDE) examined by reverse phase high performance liquid chromatography (HPLC). Apparently, PB and DDE, whose chemical structures are very different from each other, induce an identical form of cytochrome P-450 in rat liver microsomes. Similar observations have recently been reported by Lau et al. (17) using β-naphthoflavone and MC as inducers, and by Toftgurd et al. (35) using xylene and PB as inducers.

On the other hand, some xenobiotic compounds induce more than one form of cytochrome P-450 in the liver microsomes of treated rats (6, 11, 18, 20, 23, 28, 31, 34, 36–38). In addition to the major PB-inducible form of cytochrome P-450, P-450$_b$ (32) or P-450(PB-1) (13), PB seems to induce one (28, 37, 38), two (31), or three (6, 36) other similar forms of the cytochrome. MC also induces one major and another minor form, P-450$_c$ and P-450$_d$, respectively, of cytochrome P-450 in rat liver microsomes.

Phenobarbital- and 3-Methylcholanthrene-induced Synthesis of P-450(PB-1) and P-450 (MC-1) in Rat Liver

To study the mechanism of the drug-induced increase of P-450(PB-1) or P-450 (MC-1) in rat liver microsomes, the rates of synthesis of these two inducible forms of cytochrome P-450 in the livers of untreated and drug-treated rats were studied. The syntheses of a few other microsomal enzymes were also examined for comparison.

Figure 5 shows the results of an experiment, in which L-(^{3}H)leucine was intravenously injected to PB-treated rats at various time points after PB injection (14). The animals were killed 2 hr after the radioactive leucine injection. The liver microsomes were prepared, solubilized with detergents, and immunoprecipitated to determine the radioactivities incorporated into several microsomal proteins. The incorporation of the radioactive amino acid into each protein was regarded as representing the rate of its synthesis in the liver.

As shown in the figure, P-450(PB-1), P-450(MC-1), cytochrome b_5, and NADPH-cytochrome P-450 reductase (fp$_T$) accounted respectively for 0.13%, 0.11%, 0.08%, and 0.05%, respectively, of the total protein synthesis in the liver of untreated rats (time zero). However, PB administration caused a selective increase of the rate of P-450(PB-1) synthesis, which reached a peak value of 18 times the initial rate at 12 hr after PB administration. The elevated rate of P-450(PB-1) synthesis did not significantly decrease until 24 hr. The rate of fp$_T$ synthesis increased 2-fold at 6 hr and 3-fold at 12 hr after PB administration, but returned to the original level at 24 hr. The syntheses of P-450(MC-1) and cytochrome b_5 were not affected by PB at all.

The effect of MC administration on the synthesis of microsomal enzymes is shown

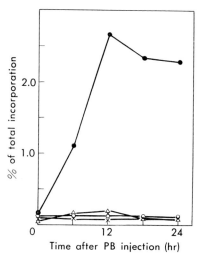

FIG. 5.   Effect of PB on the incorporation of L-(^{3}H)leucine into microsomal proteins in rat liver (*14*). PB was injected intraperitoneally to rats at time zero. L-(^{3}H)
leucine was then injected intravenously to the animals at the time points shown,
and the animals were killed 2 hr later. The incorporation of L-(^{3}H)leucine into
P-450(PB-1) (●), P-450(MC-1) (○), cytochrome b_5 (×), and fp$_T$ (△) were determined, and are expressed here as their percentages of the radioactive leucine
incorporation into total liver protein.

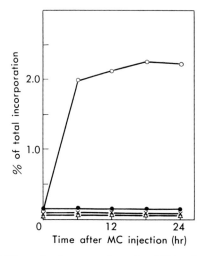

FIG. 6.   Effect of MC on the incorporation of L-(^{3}H)leucine into microsomal
proteins (*14*). MC was injected intraperitoneally to rats at time zero. The incorporation of L-(^{3}H)leucine into microsomal proteins in the livers of treated
animals was determined and is shown as described in the legend to Fig. 5.

in Fig. 6 (*14*). The rate of P-450(MC-1) synthesis increased more than 20 times the
original rate at 6 hr after MC administration, and maintained this level until 24 hr.
The rates of P-450(PB-1), cytochrome b_5, and fp$_T$ syntheses were not affected.

    The selective induction of P-450(PB-1) and P-450(MC-1) syntheses by the drugs
was also confirmed by immunochemical analyses of the nascent peptides discharged

from isolated ribosomes and the *in vitro* translation products of isolated polysomes or liver RNA (*14*). The specificity of the analysis of nascent peptides or *in vitro* translation products by immunoprecipitation was confirmed by competition experiments using authentic antigens.

The observed highly selective increase of the syntheses of P-450(PB-1) and P-450 (MC-1) by PB and MC, respectively, was in accord with the reports from other laboratories (*1,3,24*), and explains selective induction of these particular forms of cytochrome P-450 by the drugs (*13*).

Turnover of P-450(PB-1) and P-450(MC-1) in Rat Liver

The *in vivo* label experiment with a radioactive amino acid indicated a remarkable increase in the synthesis of the two inducible forms of microsomal cytochrome P-450 in the livers of drug-treated animals. Since the concentration of each form of cytochrome P-450 in liver microsomes is dependent on an equilibrium between its synthesis and degradation, we also studied the turnover rates of P-450(PB-1) and P-450(MC-1) in the livers of untreated and drug-treated rats to examine whether the inducers affect the turnover of the microsomal proteins. Intraperitoneal injection of sodium (^{14}C)bicarbonate was used to label the protein portion of the cytochrome, whereas intravenous injection of δ-amino-(^{14}C)levulinic acid was used to label the heme portion. The turnover rates of two other microsomal proteins, cytochrome b_5 and fp$_T$, were also determined.

Figures 7 and 8 (*29*) show the results of the turnover experiments with untreated and PB-treated rats, respectively. The half-lives of the microsomal proteins were

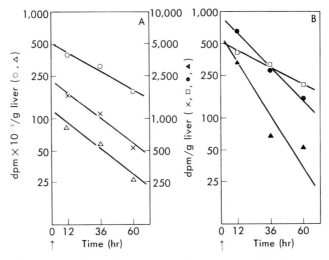

FIG. 7. Decay of specific radioactivities of microsomal proteins in the livers of untreated rats (*29*). Sodium (^{14}C)bicarbonate was intraperitoneally injected to a group of rats at time zero (arrow), and three rats were killed at the time points indicated to determine the specific radioactivities per gram liver of (A) liver homogenate (○), microsomes (△), and fp$_T$ (×), (B) cytochrome b_5 (□), P-450 (PB-1) (●), and P-450(MC-1) (▲). Each data point shown represents the average of two sets of experiments.

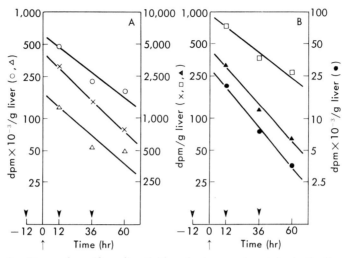

FIG. 8.   Decay of specific radioactivities of microsomal proteins in the livers of
PB-treated rats (29). The experimental procedures and symbols are the same as
described in the legend to Fig. 7 except that the animals received intraperitoneal
injections of PB at 12 hr before the injection of sodium (^{14}C)bicarbonate (arrow),
and also at 12 hr and 36 hr after the labeling (arrow heads).

TABLE I.   Half-lives of Microsomal Proteins in the Livers of Untreated and PB-treated Rats (29)

Proteins	Untreated rats		PB-treated rats
	Protein	Heme	Protein
	half-lives (hr)		
Total microsomes	35	20	25
P-450(PB-1)	25	15	20
P-450(MC-1)	15	15	20
fp_T	35	—	25
Cytochrome b_5	50	40	30

graphically determined from the figures, and are summarized in Table I (29). The
half-lives of the heme portions of P-450(PB-1), P-450(MC-1), and cytochrome b_5 in
the livers of untreated animals (29) are also listed in the table.

The turnover of the protein portions of P-450(PB-1) and P-450(MC-1) in the
livers of untreated rats was significantly faster than that of total microsomal protein as
well as those of two other microsomal membrane-bound proteins, fp_T and cytochrome
b_5. The high turnover rates of these two drug-inducible forms of cytochrome P-450
agree with their rapid increases in response to the administration of the drugs (Figs.
1 and 2), but their turnover rates were not significantly affected by the administration
of PB. The rapid increase of P-450(PB-1) in the liver microsomes of the drug-treated
rats seems to be exclusively due to an increased synthesis.

The turnover rates of P-450(PB-1) and P-450(MC-1) in the livers of untreated
rats differed, indicating that the various forms of cytochrome P-450 in liver microsomes turn over at different rates. Recently, Parkinson et al. (22) also determined the

half-lives of three immunologically distinguishable forms of microsomal cytochrome P-450 in the livers of polychlorinated biphenyl-treated rats. They obtained an identical half-life for both PB-inducible form, P-450$_{b+e}$, and MC-inducible form, P-450$_c$, but the turnover rate of another form, P-450$_a$, was clearly different from the drug-inducible forms. The half-life of P-450$_{b+e}$ reported by Parkinson and his colleagues (22), 37 hr, is significantly longer than our value for the corresponding form of the cytochrome, P-450(PB-1) (Table I). Gasser *et al.* (8) also reported the half-life of P-450$_b$ in the liver of PB-treated rats, and their value of 19 hr is close to ours. These differences among the reported half-lives of the major PB-inducible form of cytochrome P-450 in rat liver may be due to different strains or physiological conditions of the animals.

The half-life of the total heme of rat liver microsomes was about 20 hr (Table I). Since the half-life of the heme of cytochrome b_5, another major hemoprotein in the microsomes, was 40 hr, the mean half-life of the heme of various forms of cytochrome P-450 in rat liver microsomes must be shorter than 20 hr. The heme of P-450(PB-1) seems to be turning over faster than its protein moiety, suggesting that the heme of P-450(PB-1) is dissociable from its protein moiety. Although P-450(MC-1) showed an identical turnover rate for its protein and heme portions (Table I), there is evidence for reversible dissociation and association of heme with the protein moiety of microsomal cytochrome P-450 *in vivo* (5, 30). Apparently, heme is not tightly associated with the protein moiety of cytochrome P-450.

The role of heme in the induction of cytochrome P-450 in the liver is not yet clarified. There is evidence that the induction of microsomal cytochrome P-450 by PB is dependent on the availability of heme (9), and one report (27) suggested the regulation of the biosynthesis of the protein moiety of a PB-inducible form of cytochrome P-450 by the level of heme pool in the cell. However, the incorporation of heme to newly synthesized cytochrome P-450 does not seem to be tightly coupled with the synthesis of the protein moiety (30).

Induction of P-450(PB-1) mRNA in Rat Liver by Phenobarbital and 1,1-Di(p-chlorophenyl)-2,2-dichloroethylene

Since the turnover rate of P-450(PB-1) in the liver was not affected by PB administration to rats, the drug-induced rapid increase of this particular form of cytochrome P-450 must be explained by its stimulated synthesis. Recent progress in the cloning of cDNAs for the mRNAs or the genes of various forms of cytochrome P-450 has enabled us to determine the amounts of the mRNAs of particular forms of cytochrome P-450 by their hybridization with suitable cDNA probes. We determined the amounts of P-450(PB-1) mRNA in the RNA samples prepared from drug-treated rats by both the cell-free translation of the samples and the hybridization using a cloned cDNA to P-450(PB-1) mRNA, pcP-450pb$_4$ (7).

A single intraperitoneal injection of PB or DDE was given to rats to induce P-450 (PB-1), and RNA was prepared from the livers of the drug-treated animals at various time points after the drug administration. Figure 9 (19) shows the results of the cell-free translation of total liver RNA samples in reticulocyte lysate. Poly(A)RNA was also prepared from the total liver RNA, and P-450(PB-1) mRNA was determined by the

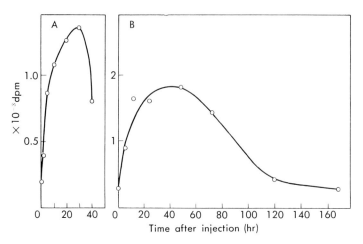

Fɪɢ. 9. Synthesis of P-450(PB-1) peptide by cell-free translation of liver total RNA from PB-treated and DDE-treated rats (*19*). PB (A) or DDE (B) was intraperitoneally injected to a group of rats at time zero, and three animals were killed at each time point shown to prepare total RNA from their livers. The *in vitro* translation of the RNA was carried out in a reticulocyte lysate using L-(^{35}S) methionine to label the synthesized peptides. P-450(PB-1) peptide was immunoprecipitated from the translation products by specific antibodies, and detected by fluorography after SDS-polyacrylamide gel electrophoresis of the immunoprecipitates. The radioactive band corresponding to P-450(PB-1) peptide was cut out from the dried gel, and the radioactivity was determined as shown.

dot hybridization of the poly(A)RNA samples using a cloned cDNA to P-450(PB-1) mRNA as shown in Fig. 10 (*19*).

In the experiment shown in Fig. 9, rat liver RNA was translated *in vitro* with L-(^{35}S)methionine to label the synthesized peptides, and the translation products were immunoprecipitated to isolate P-450(PB-1) peptides. The immunoprecipitates were analyzed by SDS-polyacrylamide gel electrophoresis and fluorography, and the radioactive band corresponding to P-450(PB-1) was cut out from the dried gel to determine the radioactivity. Judging from the amounts of the *in vitro* synthesized P-450(PB-1) peptide, P-450(PB-1) mRNA increased rapidly after the PB administration, attaining a peak value at 20–30 hr, which was about 8 times higher than the initial level at time zero, and then rapidly declined (Fig. 9A). In DDE-treated rats (Fig. 9B), the peak of P-450(PB-1) mRNA was at 40–60 hr after the administration of the chemical, and its decline was slower than PB-treated rats.

Quantitation of P-450(PB-1) mRNA by dot hybridization was carried out as described by Brooker and O'Connar (*2*). Various amounts of poly(A)RNA from the livers of PB-treated or DDE-treated rats were applied to a nitrocellulose filter, and hybridized with the ^{32}P-labeled cDNA probe prepared by nick-translation of the insert of pcP-450pb$_4$. The hybridized spots were detected by autoradiography, and their radioactivities were counted (Fig. 10). As can be seen, the time courses of the increase and decline of P-450(PB-1) mRNA determined by the hybridization assay were essentially the same as those determined by the cell-free translation assay. The observed rapid and large increase of P-450(PB-1) mRNA induced by a single administration of PB

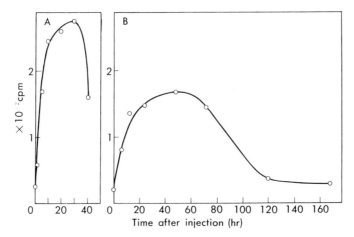

F_{IG}. 10.   Quantitation of P-450(PB-1) mRNA in rat liver RNA by dot hybridization using cloned P-450(PB-1) cDNA (*19*). Poly(A)RNA was prepared from the livers of PB-treated rats (A) or DDE-treated rats (B) at various time points as shown after drug administration at time zero. The amounts of P-450(PB-1) mRNA in the poly(A)RNA were determined by dot hybridization using cloned P-450(PB-1) cDNA as the hybridization probe. The spots of poly(A)RNA samples hybridized with the ^{32}P-labeled cDNA probe were detected by autoradiography, and the radioactivities of the spots are shown.

is generally in agreement with the reports from other laboratories (*1, 3, 10*). The hybridization assay also confirmed that PB and DDE induced an identical form of cytochrome P-450 in rat liver.

We can conclude that various xenobiotic compounds induce particular molecular species of cytochrome P-450 in liver microsomes by increasing their translatable mRNAs in the cell. How a wide variety of chemical compounds rapidly and selectively increase the amounts of the mRNAs of one or a few particular molecular species of cytochrome P-450 is an important and urgent problem requiring clarification.

Acknowledgment

The author wishes to thank Drs. Yoshiaki Fujii-Kuriyama, Nobuhiro Harada, Shin-ichi Kuwahara, Toshiyuki Miyata, and Kazuhiro Sogawa, and Messrs. Ken-ichirou Morohashi, Hiroyuki Sadano, and Hidefumi Yoshioka for their collaboration in this study.

REFERENCES

1.   Bhat, K. S. and Padmanaban, G. Studies on the biosynthesis of cytochrome P-450 in rat liver. A probe with phenobarbital. *Arch. Biochem. Biophys.*, **198**, 110–116 (1979).
2.   Brooker, J. D. and O'Connar, R. cDNA cloning and analysis of chick embryo liver cytochrome P-450 mRNA induced by porphyrinogenic drugs. *Eur. J. Biochem.*, **129**, 325–333 (1982).
3.   Colbert, R. A., Bresnick, E., Levin, W., Ryan, D. E., and Thomas, P. E. Synthesis of liver cytochrome P-450 in a cell-free protein synthesizing system. *Biochem. Biophys. Res. Commun.*, **91**, 886–891 (1979).

4. Conney, A. H. Pharmacological implications of microsomal enzyme induction. *Pharmacol. Rev.*, **19**, 317–366 (1967).

5. Correia, M. A., Farrell, G. C., Olson, S., Wong, J. S., Schmid, R., Ortiz deMontellano, P. R., Belian, H. S., Kunze, K. L., and Mico, B. A. Cytochrome P-450 heme moiety. The specific target in drug-induced heme alkylation. *J. Biol. Chem.*, **256**, 5466–5470 (1981).

6. Dannan, G. A., Guengerich, F. P., Kaminsky, L. S., and Aust, S. D. Regulation of cytochrome P-450. Immunochemical quantitation of eight isozymes in liver microsomes of rats treated with polybromominated biphenyl congeners. *J. Biol. Chem.*, **258**, 1282–1288 (1983).

7. Fujii-Kuriyama, Y., Mizukami, Y., Kawajiri, K., Sogawa, K., and Muramatsu, M. Primary structure of a cytochrome P-450: coding nucleotide sequence of phenobarbital-inducible cytochrome P-450 cDNA from rat liver. *Proc. Natl. Acad. Sci. U.S.*, **79**, 2793–2797 (1982).

8. Gasser, R., Hauri, H. P., and Meyer, U. A. The turnover of cytochrome P-450$_b$. *FEBS Lett.*, **147**, 239–242 (1982).

9. Giger, U. and Meyer, U. A. Effect of succinylacetone on heme and cytochrome P-450 synthesis in hepatocyte culture. *FEBS Lett.*, **153**, 335–338 (1983).

10. Gonzalez, F. J. and Kasper, C. B. Cloning of DNA complementary to rat liver NADPH-cytochrome *c* oxidoreductase and cytochrome P-450$_b$ mRNAs. *J. Biol. Chem.*, **257**, 5962–5968 (1982).

11. Guengerich, F. P., Dannan, G. A., Wright, S. T., Martin, M. V., and Kaminsky, L. S. Purification and characterization of liver microsomal cytochrome P-450. Electrophoretic, catalytic, and immunochemical properties and inducibility of eight isozymes isolated from rats treated with phenobarbital or β-naphthoflavone. *Biochemistry*, **21**, 6019–6030 (1982).

12. Guengerich, F. P., Wang, P., and Davidson, N. Estimation of isozymes of microsomal cytochrome P-450 in rats, rabbits, and humans using immunochemical staining coupled with sodium dodecyl sulfate-polyacrylamide gel electrophoresis. *Biochemistry*, **21**, 1698–1706 (1982).

13. Harada, N. and Omura, T. Selective induction of two different molecular species of cytochrome P-450 by phenobarbital and 3-methylcholanthrene. *J. Biochem.*, **89**, 237–248 (1981).

14. Harada, N. and Omura, T. Phenobarbital- and 3-methylcholanthrene-induced synthesis of two different molecular species of microsomal cytochrome P-450 in rat liver. *J. Biochem.*, **93**, 1361–1373 (1983).

15. Hunnego, N. J. and Harrison, D. L. Metabolism of DDE, DDD, and DDT in sheep. *N. Z. J. Agr. Res.*, **14**, 406–416 (1971).

16. Kuwahara, S., Harada, N., Yoshioka, H., Miyata, T., and Omura, T. Purification and characterization of four forms of cytochrome P-450 from liver microsomes of phenobarbital-treated and 3-methylcholanthrene-treated rats. *J. Biochem.*, **95**, 703–714 (1984).

17. Lau, P. P., Pickett, C. B., Lu, A.Y.H., and Strobel, H. W. Comparison of cytochrome P-450 with high activity toward benzo(a)pyrene purified from liver microsomes of β-naphthoflavone- and 3-methylcholanthrene-treated rats. *Arch. Biochem. Biophys.*, **218**, 472–477 (1982).

18. Luster, M. I., Lawson, L. D., Linko, P., and Goldstein, J. A. Immunochemical evidence for two 3-methylcholanthrene-inducible forms of cytochrome P-448 in rat liver microsomes using a double-antibody radioimmunoassay procedure. *Mol. Pharmacol.*, **23**, 252–257 (1983).

19. Morohashi, K., Yoshioka, H., Sogawa, K., Fujii-Kuriyama, Y., and Omura, T. Induction of mRNA coding for phenobarbital-inducible form of microsomal cytochrome P-450 in rat liver by administration of 1,1-di(p-chlorophenyl)-2,2-dichloroethylene and phenobarbital. *J. Biochem.*, **95**, 949–957 (1984).

20. Morville, A. L., Thomas, P. E., Levin, W., Reik, L., Ryan, D. E., Raphael, C., and Adesnik, M. The accumulation of distinct mRNAs for the immunochemically related cytochrome P-450$_c$ and P-450$_d$ in rat liver following 3-methylcholanthrene treatment. *J. Biol. Chem.*, **258**, 3901–3906 (1983).

21. Newman, S. L., Barwick, J. L., Elshourbagy, N. A., and Guzelian, P. S. Measurement of the metabolism of cytochrome P-450 in cultured hepatocytes by a quantitative and specific immunochemical method. *Biochem. J.*, **204**, 281–290 (1982).

22. Parkinson, A., Thomas, P. E., Ryan, D. E., and Levin, W. The *in vivo* turnover of rat liver microsomal epoxide hydrolase and both the apoprotein and heme moieties of specific cytochrome P-450 isozymes. *Arch. Biochem. Biophys.*, **225**, 216–236 (1983).

23. Parkinson, A., Safe, S. H., Robertson, L. W., Thomas, P. E., Ryan, D. E., Reik, L. M., and Levin, W. Immunochemical quantitation of cytochrome P-450 isozymes and epoxide hydrolase in liver microsomes from polychlorinated or polybrominated biphenyl-treated rats. *J. Biol. Chem.*, **258**, 5967–5976 (1983).

24. Phillips, I. R., Shephard, E. A., Mitani, F., and Rabin, B. R. Induction by phenobarbital of the mRNA for a specific variant of rat liver microsomal cytochrome P-450. *Biochem. J.*, **196**, 839–851 (1981).

25. Phillips, I. R., Shephard, E. A., Bayney, R. M., Pike, S. F., Rabin, B. R., Heath, R., and Carter, N. Induction and repression of the major phenobarbital-induced cytochrome P-450 measured by radioimmunoassay. *Biochem. J.*, **212**, 55–64 (1983).

26. Pickett, C. B., Jeter, R. L., Morin, J., and Lu, A.Y.H. Electroimmunochemical quantitation of cytochrome P-450, cytochrome P-448, and epoxide hydrolase in rat liver microsomes. *J. Biol. Chem.*, **256**, 8815–8820 (1981).

27. Ravishankar, H. and Padmanaban, G. Effect of cobalt chloride and 3-amino-1,2,4-triazole on the induction of cytochrome P-450 synthesis by phenobarbital in rat liver. *Arch. Biochem. Biophys.*, **225**, 16–24 (1983).

28. Ryan, D. E., Thomas, P. E., and Levin, W. Purification and characterization of a minor form of hepatic microsomal cytochrome P-450 from rats treated with polychlorinated biphenyls. *Arch. Biochem. Biophys.*, **216**, 272–288 (1982).

29. Sadano, H. and Omura, T. Turnover of two drug-inducible forms of microsomal cytochrome P-450 in rat liver. *J. Biochem.*, **93**, 1375–1383 (1983).

30. Sadano, H. and Omura, T. Reversible transfer of heme between different molecular species of microsome-bound cytochrome P-450 in rat liver. *Biochem. Biophys. Res. Commun.*, **116**, 1013–1019 (1983).

31. Sakai, H., Hino, Y., and Minakami, S. Three immunoidentical cytochrome P-450 from liver microsomes of phenobarbital-treated rats. *Biochem. J.*, **215**, 83–89 (1983).

32. Thomas, P. E., Korzeniowsky, K., Ryan, D.E., and Levin, W. Preparation of monospecific antibodies against two forms of rat liver cytochrome P-450 and quantitation of these antigens in microsomes. *Arch. Biochem. Biophys.*, **192**, 524–532 (1979).

33. Thomas, P. E., Reik, L. M., Ryan, D. E., and Levin, W. Regulation of three forms of cytochrome P-450 and epoxide hydrolase in rat liver microsomes. *J. Biol. Chem.*, **256**, 1044–1052 (1981).

34. Thomas, P. E., Reik, L. M., Ryan, D. E., and Levin, W. Induction of two immunochemically related rat liver cytochrome P-450 isozymes, cytochromes P-450$_c$ and P-450$_d$, by structurally diverse xenobiotics. *J. Biol. Chem.*, **258**, 4590–4598 (1983).

35. Toftgurd, R., Halpert, J., and Gustafsson, J. A. Xylene induces a cytochrome P-450 isozyme in rat liver similar to the major isozyme induced by phenobarbital. *Mol. Pharmacol.*, **23**, 265–271 (1984).
36. Vlasuk, G. P., Ghrayeb, J., Ryan, D. E., Reik, L., Thomas, P. E., Levin, W., and Walz, Jr., F. G. Multiplicity, strain differences, and topology of phenobarbital-induced cytochrome P-450 in rat liver microsomes. *Biochemistry*, **21**, 789–798 (1982).
37. Vlasuk, G. P., Ryan, D. E., Thomas, P. E., Levin, W., and Walz, Jr., F. G. Polypeptide patterns of hepatic microsomes from Long-Evans rats treated with different xenobiotics. *Biochemistry*, **21**, 6288–6292 (1982).
38. Waxman, D. J. and Walsh, C. Phenobarbital-induced rat liver cytochrome P-450. Purification and characterization of two closely related isozyme forms. *J. Biol. Chem.*, **257**, 10446–10457 (1982).
39. Yoshioka, H., Miyata, T., and Omura, T. Induction of a phenobarbital-inducible form of cytochrome P-450 in rat liver microsomes by 1,1-di(p-chlorophenyl)-2,2-dichloroethylene. *J. Biochem.*, **95**, 937–947 (1984).

MOLECULAR MULTIPLICITY AND GENE STRUCTURE OF MICROSOMAL CYTOCHROME P-450 IN RAT LIVER

Yoshiaki Fujii-Kuriyama,[*1] Kazuhiro Sogawa,[*1] Yuzuru Mizukami,[*1,*4]
Yorimasa Suwa,[*1] Masami Muramatsu,[*2] Kaname Kawajiri,[*3]
Osamu Gotoh,[*3] and Yusaku Tagashira[*3]

*Department of Biochemistry, Cancer Institute,[*1] Department of Biochemistry,
Faculty of Medicine, University of Tokyo,[*2] and Department of
Biochemistry, Saitama Cancer Center Research Institute[*3]*

cDNA clones of phenobarbital (PB)-inducible cytochrome P-450
and a methylcholanthrene-inducible one were identified by hybridization-
selected translation assay. From analyses of coding nucleotide sequences
in these cloned DNA, the primary amino acid sequences for two forms
of PB-inducible cytochrome P-450 (P-450b and e) and one form of
methylcholanthrene-inducible cytochrome P-450 (P-450d) were deduced.

Structural comparison of these amino acid sequences, together with
those of other forms of cytochrome P-450 determined from protein analysis clearly showed two highly conserved regions consisting of approximately 20 amino acids. One of these is proposed as the heme binding site.

Using the cloned P-450b cDNA as a probe, six independent genomic
clones were isolated from a rat gene library and one was subjected to
structural analysis. The characteristic of the gene structure for PB-
inducible cytochrome P-450 is reported.

Cytochrome P-450, a class of terminal exidases of a microsomal NADPH-dependent
electron transport pathway, is involved in the biotransformation of a wide variety of
structurally unrelated compounds, including steroids, fatty acids, various kinds of
drugs, hydrocarbons, and chemical carcinogens. It has now been well established that
this unusually broad substrate specificity of the system relates to the presence of multiple
molecular forms of cytochrome P-450. Each form has a rather broad and different substrate specificity, and sometimes shows overlapping specificity with others (*12, 21, 25*).

Some forms of these cytochrome P-450's are inducible enzymes: Administration
of a certain drug to animals induces the synthesis of a specific form of cytochrome
P-450. Among inducers are phenobarbital (PB), 3-methylcholanthrene (MC), isosafrole,
polychlorinated biphenyl, β-naphthoflavon, pregnenolone-16α-carbonitile and so on.

Studies at a gene or DNA level of cytochrome P-450 using recombinant DNA
technology may be most informative for understanding the molecular events under-
lying the multiplicity and the selective drug induction of the cytochrome.

[*1] Kami-Ikebukuro 1-37-1, Toshima-ku, Tokyo 170, Japan (藤井義明, 十川和博, 水上　譲, 諏訪頼正).
[*2] Hongo 7-3-1, Bunkyo-ku, Tokyo 113, Japan (村松正実).
[*3] Ina-machi, Kitaadachi-gun, Saitama 362, Japan (川尻　要, 後藤　修, 田頭勇作).
[*4] Present address: Laboratory of Microbiology II, Central Research Laboratory, Meiji Seika, Ltd.

We previously cloned and sequenced cDNA's for mRNA's of PB-inducible cyto-chrome P-450 (P-450b and P-450e) and therefrom deduced their primary amino acid sequences (*9, 10*). We have also predicted the complete amino acid sequence of MC- and isosafrol-inducible cytochrome P-450 (P-450d) by sequence analysis of the cloned cDNA's (*17, 19*). This form of cytochrome P-450 has very recently also been shown to play also an important role in the metabolic activation of potent carcinogenic sub-stances such as amino acid pyrolysates (Trp P-2 and Glu P-2 *etc.*) (*18*). By comparing these sequences and others which were determined from sequence analysis of purified proteins, we have determined a conserved segment in various forms of cytochrome P-450 molecules which contain a cystein residue postulated to ligate the heme. To understand the mechanism of drug induction of cytochrome P-450, we have isolated and analyzed the genomic clones. A comparison between gene sequences of various forms of drug inducible cytochrome P-450's is now underway with special attention to the sequences of the promoter regions, upstream sequences of the transcription initiation sites. In this paper, we describe the structural characteristics of cytochrome P-450's obtained from sequence analysis of cloned cDNAs and the gene structure of a PB inducible cytochrome P-450.

cDNA Cloning of Cytochrome P-450

Administration of phenobarbital to experimental animals causes the inductive synthesis of specific forms of cytochrome P-450 (P-450b and e for rats) in the liver with concomitant increase in the corresponding cytochrome P-450 mRNA activity (*6, 7*). The mRNA was usually increased in amount from several- to 10-fold about 15 hr after the treatment with the drug. Taking advantage of this induction phenomenon, several groups including ours prepared the mRNA for the cytochrome (*1, 9*). Extracted RNA from PB-treated rats was applied on a oligo(dT)-cellulose column for isolation of poly(A)$^+$RNA and then the poly(A)$^+$RNA was centrifuged in a sucrose density gradient. The mRNA for the cytochrome P-450 gave a sedimentation velocity constant of ap-proximately 18S which suggested the mRNA length to be about 2,000 bases. The cytochrome P-450 mRNA in the peak fraction was assumed to occupy 1 to 3% of the 18S RNA fraction from the mRNA activity assayed in an *in vitro* translation system (*9*). cDNA was synthesized from this mRNA preparation by avian myeloblastosis virus (AMV) reverse transcriptase and then the cDNA was made double-stranded using the reverse transcriptase again. The ds-cDNA was inserted into pBR322 at the *Pst* I site by the GC-tailing method to transform *Escherichia coli* χ 1776.

Transformed cells harboring hybrid plasmid of a P-450 cDNA sequence were selected by both hybridization-arrested and hybridization-selected translation assay. Five positive clones were identified from among 2,000 transformants.

By essentially the same procedure as described above, we constructed and isolated the cDNA clone of MC-inducible cytochrome P-450d. In this case, poly(A)$^+$RNA was prepared from livers of MC-treated rats and we used 18S RNA fraction of this poly(A)$^+$RNA in sucrose density gradient centrifugation for the synthesis of cDNA, because this 18S RNA fraction showed the highest mRNA activity for MC-inducible cyto-chrome P-450 in the *in vitro* translation system of rabbit reticulocyte lysates (*19*).

Sequence Analysis of Cloned cDNA's for Cytochrome P-450

The amino acid sequences of two forms of PB-inducible and one form of MC-inducible cytochrome P-450 were determined by sequence analysis of the cloned cDNA's. These are shown in Figs. 1 and 2. By comparison with the sequence of 21 N-terminal amino acids obtained from analysis of the purified protein, the upper sequence in Fig. 1 was found to code for cytochrome P-450b as designated by Botelho *et al.* (*3*); this is involved in the metabolic activation of aflatoxin B_1 (*20*). The lower sequence has recently been revealed to correspond to the mRNA for cytochrome P-450e, a minor form of PB-inducible cytochrome P-450 (*26*).

At approximately the same time that the primary amino acid sequences of PB-inducible cytochrome P-450 were identified, Haniu *et al.* achieved the sequence analysis of the purified protein of *Pseudomonas putida* P-450cam (*14*). We were therefore able to compare these sequences and determine two highly homologous regions between rat cytochrome P-450 and bacterial cytochrome P-450cam (Fig. 3) (*11*). One region, called HR1 is located near the NH_2-terminus of the cytochrome P-450 molecule (from Val[142] Arg[158] for rat cytochrome P-450 and from Leu[125] to Arg[141] for *Pseudomonas* cytochrome P-450cam), while the other (HR2) is near the COOH-terminus (from Phe[429] to Leu[448] for rat P-450 and from Phe[348] to Val[367] for *Pseudomonas* P-450cam). Since the optical and magnetic properties of various P-450 species are very similar, the primary as well as the secondary and tertiary structures around the heme binding sites are expected to be well conserved even in remotely related P-450's. Moreover, there is accumulating evidence of coordination of a cysteine residue to the heme of cytochrome P-450 (*13*). Interestingly, both HR1 and HR2 contain a cysteine near the center of the homologous region. Which cysteine residue of these two homologous regions might function as the 5th coordinate to the heme? Dus and his coworkers isolated a peptide fragment that retains the heme after cleaving a purified rabbit P-450 LM2 by cyanogen bromide treatment and determined the amino acid composition of the heme peptide (*8*). Since the amino acid composition of rat P-450b hemepeptide is not available and since rabbit P-450LM2 is an equivalent protein to rat P-450b from the aspects of drug-inducibility, substrate specificity, overall amino acid composition and N-terminal sequences, we scrutinized the primary amino acid sequence of P-450b for a local peptide fragment of about 40 amino acids which gives an amino acid composition close to that of the heme peptide from rabbit P-450LM2.

The amino acid composition of the peptide (Pro[428]-Asp[467]) which covers HR2 shows a similarity closer to that of the isolated heme peptide than to that of the peptide around HR1 (*9*). In the amino acid sequence of P-450d we can easily find local sequences corresponding to HR1 and HR2.

Figure 4 summarizes the comparison of the amino acid sequences in these two conserved regions of six molecular species of cytochrome P-450 so far analyzed. The sequence of cytochrome P-450 of porcine adrenal 21 hydroxylase is taken from the partial amino acid sequence reported by Haniu *et al.* (*15*).

The cysteine residue near the center of HR2 is common to all the P-450 sequences, whereas the cysteine in the middle of HR1 is replaced by histidine residue in the P-450d sequence. This cysteine is also replaced by tyrosine in the P-450c sequence (unpublished observation by Sogawa *et al.*). Considering this together with the fact that HR2 is more

```
                                        10                                        20
Met Glu Pro Thr Ile Leu Leu Leu Leu Ala Leu Leu Val Gly Phe Leu Leu Leu Leu Val Arg Gly His Pro Lys
                                        TTG CTC CTC CTT GCT CTC CTC GTG GGC TTC TTG TTA CTC TTA GTC AGG GGA CAC CCA AAG

                         30                                        40                                     50
Ser Arg Gly Asn Phe Pro Pro Gly Pro Arg Pro Leu Pro Leu Leu Gly Asn Leu Leu Gln Leu Asp Arg Gly Gly
TCC CGT GGC AAC TTC CCA CCA GGA CCT CGT CCC CTT CCC CTC TTG GGG AAC CTC CTG CAG TTG GAC AGA GGG GGC
                                            ↑──────→ pcP-450 pb4
                                                              70
Leu Leu Asn Ser Phe Met Gln Leu Arg Glu Lys Tyr Gly Asp Val Phe Thr Val His Leu Gly Pro Arg Pro Val
CTC CTC AAT TCC TTC ATG CAG CTT CGA GAA AAA TAT GGA GAT GTG TTC ACA GTA CAC CTG GGA CCA AGG CCT GTG
     ↑──────→ pcP-450 pb2
                                                    90                                        100
Val Met Leu Cys Gly Thr Asp Thr Ile Lys Glu Ala Leu Val Gly Gln Ala Glu Asp Phe Ser Gly Arg Gly Thr
GTC ATG CTA TGT GGG ACA GAC ACC ATA AAG GAG GCT CTG GTG GGC CAA GCT GAG GAT TTC TCT GGT CGG GGA ACA

                                        110                                        120
Ile Ala Val Ile Glu Pro Ile Phe Lys Glu Tyr Gly Val Ile Phe Ala Asn Gly Glu Arg Trp Lys Ala Leu Arg
ATC GCT GTG ATT GAG CCA ATC TTC AAG GAA TAT GGT GTG ATC TTT GCC AAT GGG GAA CGC TGG AAG GCC CTT CGG

                     130                                        140                                     150
Arg Phe Ser Leu Ala Thr Met Arg Asp Phe Gly Met Gly Lys Arg Ser Val Glu Glu Arg Ile Gln Glu Glu Ala
CGA TTC TCT CTG GCT ACC ATG AGA GAC TTT GGG ATG GGA AAG AGG AGT GTG GAA GAA CGG ATT CAG GAG GAA GCC

                                        160                                        170
Gln Cys Leu Val Glu Glu Leu Arg Lys Ser Gln Gly Ala Pro Leu Asp Pro Thr Phe Leu Phe Gln Cys Ile Thr
CAA TGT TTG GTG GAG GAA CTG CGG AAA TCC CAG GGA GCC CCA CTG GAT CCC ACC TTC CTC TTC CAG TGC ATC ACA

                     180                                        190                                     200
Ala Asn Ile Ile Cys Ser Ile Val Phe Gly Glu Arg Phe Asp Tyr Thr Asp Arg Gln Phe Leu Arg Leu Leu Glu
GCC AAC ATC ATC TGC TCC ATT GTG TTT GGA GAG CGC TTT GAC TAC ACA GAC CGC CAG TTC CTG CGC CTG TTG GAG
                                    ↑──────→ pcP-450 pb1
                                                    220
Leu Phe Tyr Arg Thr Phe Ser Leu Leu Ser Ser Phe Ser Ser Gln Val Phe Glu Phe Phe Ser Gly Phe Leu Lys
CTG TTC TAC CGG ACC TTT TCC CTC CTA AGT TCA TTC TCC AGC CAG GTG TTT GAG TTC TTC TCT GGG TTC CTG AAA

                     230                                        240                                     250
Tyr Phe Pro Gly Ala His Arg Gln Ile Ser Lys Asn Leu Gln Glu Ile Leu Asp Tyr Ile Gly His Ile Val Glu
TAC TTT CCT GGT GCC CAC AGA CAA ATC TCC AAA AAC CTC CAG GAA ATC CTC GAT TAC ATT GGC CAT ATT GTG GAG

                                        260                                        270
Lys His Arg Ala Thr Leu Asp Pro Ser Ala Pro Arg Asp Phe Ile Asp Thr Tyr Leu Leu Arg Met Glu Lys Glu
AAG CAC AGG GCC ACC TTA GAC CCA AGC GCT CCA CGA GAC TTC ATC GAC ACT TAC CTT CTG CGC ATG GAG AAG GAG

                 280                                        290                                        300
Lys Ser Asn His His Thr Glu Phe His His Glu Asn Leu Met Ile Ser Leu Leu Ser Leu Phe Phe Ala Gly Thr
AAG TCG AAC CAC CAC ACA GAG TTC CAT CAT GAG AAC CTC ATG ATC TCC CTG CTC TCT CTC TTC TTT GCT GGC ACT

        Gly                                                                  Thr Val
Glu Thr Ser Ser Thr Thr Leu Arg Tyr Gly Phe Leu Leu Met Leu Lys Tyr Pro His Val Ala Glu Lys Val Gln
GAG ACC AGC AGC ACC ACA CTC CGC TAT GGT TTC CTG CTG ATG CTC AAG TAC CCC CAT GTC GCA GAG AAA GTC CAA
        G                                         C                                   A   T

            330                         Pro      Ser 340                  Thr                 350
Lys Glu Ile Asp Gln Val Ile Gly Ser His Arg Leu Pro Thr Leu Asp Asp Arg Ser Lys Met Pro Tyr Thr Asp
AAG GAG ATT GAT CAG GTG ATC GGC TCA CAC CGG CTA CCA ACC CTT GAT GAC CGC AGT AAA ATG CCA TAC ACT GAT
                                T        T    A   C        T              T   T  CC

Ala Val Ile His Glu Ile Gln Arg Phe Ser Asp Leu Val Pro Ile Gly Val Pro His Arg Val Thr Lys Asp Thr
GCA GTT ATC CAC GAG ATT CAG AGG TTT TCA GAT CTT GTC CCT ATT GGA GTA CCA CAC AGA GTC ACC AAA GAC ACC
    C        pcP-450 pb2 ←──────↑

                                        390                                        400
Met Phe Arg Gly Tyr Leu Leu Pro Lys Asn Thr Glu Val Tyr Pro Ile Leu Ser Ser Ala Leu His Asp Pro Gln
ATG TTC CGA GGG TAC CTG CTT CCC AAG AAC ACT GAA GTG TAC CCC ATC CTG AGT TCA GCT CTC CAT GAC CCA CAG

                                        410                                        420
Tyr Phe Asp His Pro Asp Ser Phe Asn Pro Glu His Phe Leu Asp Ala Asn Gly Ala Leu Lys Lys Ser Glu Ala
TAC TTT GAC CAC CCA GAC AGC TTC AAT CCT GAA CAC TTC CTG GAT GCC AAT GGG GCA CTG AAA AAG AGT GAA GCT

            430                                        440                                        450
Phe Met Pro Phe Ser Thr Gly Lys Arg Ile Cys Leu Gly Glu Gly Ile Ala Arg Asn Glu Leu Phe Leu Phe Phe
TTC ATG CCC TTC TCC ACA GGA AAG CGC ATT TGT CTT GGC GAA GGC ATT GCC CGA AAT GAA TTG TTC CTC TTC TTC

                                        460                                        470
Thr Thr Ile Leu Gln Asn Phe Ser Val Ser Ser His Leu Ala Pro Lys Asp Ile Asp Leu Thr Pro Lys Glu Ser
ACC ACC ATC CTC CAG AAC TTC TCT GTG TCA AGC CAT TTG GCT CCC AAG GAC ATT GAC CTC ACG CCC AAG GAG AGT

            480                                        490
Gly Ile Gly Lys Ile Pro Pro Thr Tyr Gln Ile Cys Phe Ser Ala Arg
GGC ATT GGA AAA ATA CCT CCA ACG TAC CAG ATC TGC TTC TCA GCT CGG TGA TCC GGC TGA GGC AGC CAG GTG CCC

CAG TTC TGT TGG GAA TGG CCT CAT GTT TCT GCC TCT GGG GGA CCT GCT GAA AAC CAG GCT CCA AGG CCA CTG CTC

CAC ATC T.. ... ... ...
```

FIG. 1. The coding nucleotide sequence of rat PB-inducible cytochrome P-450 cDNA and its corresponding amino acid sequence. Vertical arrows indicate the start or end of the cloned cDNAs. The nucleotide sequences of pcP-450pbl and -4 (P-450b cDNA) are completely consistent with each other in their overlapping nucleotides. The nucleotide substitutions in pcP-450pb2 (P-450e cDNA) are shown below the corresponding nucleotide of the sequence of pcP-450pbl and -4. The resulting amino acid replacements are shown above the corresponding ones in the amino acid sequence.

```
                                                             - AC CCT TCA GTC GTA CAG

                                 10                                    20
Met Ala Phe Ser Gln Tyr Ile Ser Leu Ala Pro Glu Leu Leu Leu Ala Thr Ala Ile Phe Cys Leu Val Phe Trp
ATG GCG TTC TCC CAG TAT ATC TCC TTA GCC CCA GAG CTG CTA CTG GCC ACT GCC ATC TTC TGT TTA GTG TTC TGG

                                 30                                    40                          50
Val Leu Arg Gly Thr Arg Thr Gln Val Pro Lys Gly Leu Lys Ser Pro Pro Gly Pro Trp Gly Leu Pro Phe Ile
GTG TTG AGA GGC ACA AGG ACC CAG GTT CCC AAA GGT CTG AAG AGT CCT CCC GGA CCC TGG GGC TTG CCC TTC ATT

Gly His Met Leu Thr Leu Gly Lys Asn Pro His Leu Ser Leu Thr Lys Leu Ser Gln Gln Tyr Gly Asp Val Leu
GGG CAC ATG CTG ACC CTG GGG AAG AAC CCA CAC CTA TCT CTG ACA AAG CTG AGT CAG CAG TAT GGC GAC GTG CTG

                                 80                                    90                         100
Gln Ile Arg Ile Gly Ser Thr Pro Val Val Val Leu Ser Gly Leu Asn Thr Ile Lys Gln Ala Leu Val Lys Gln
CAG ATC CGC ATT GGC TCC ACA CCC GTG GTG GTG CTG AGC GGC CTG AAC ACC ATC AAG CAG GCC CTA GTG AAG CAG

Gly Asp Asp Phe Lys Gly Arg Pro Asp Leu Tyr Ser Phe Thr Leu Ile Thr Asn Gly Lys Ser Met Thr Phe Asn
GGG GAT GAC TTC AAA GGC CGG CCA GAC CTC TAC AGC TTC ACA CTT ATC ACT AAT GGC AAG AGC ATG ACT TTC AAC

                                130                                   140                         150
Pro Asp Ser Gly Pro Val Trp Ala Ala Arg Arg Arg Leu Ala Gln Asp Ala Leu Lys Ser Phe Ser Ile Ala Ser
CCA GAC TCT GGA CCG GTC TGG GCT GCC CGC CGG CGC CTG GCC CAG GAT GCC CTG AAG AGT TTC TCC ATA GCC TCA

Asp Pro Thr Ser Val Ser Ser Cys Tyr Leu Glu Glu His Val Ser Lys Glu Ala Asn His Leu Ile Ser Lys Phe
GAC CCC ACA TCA GTA TCC TCT TGC TAC TTG GAG GAG CAC GTG AGC AAA GAG GCT AAC CAT CTA ATC AGC AAG TTC

                                180                                   190                         200
Gln Lys Leu Met Ala Glu Val Gly His Phe Glu Pro Val Asn Gln Val Val Glu Ser Val Ala Asn Val Ile Gly
CAG AAG CTG ATG GCA GAG GTT GGC CAC TTC GAA CCA GTC AAC CAG GTG GTG GAA TCG GTG GCT AAT GTC ATC GGA

                                210                                   220
Ala Met Cys Phe Gly Lys Asn Phe Pro Arg Lys Ser Glu Glu Met Leu Asn Leu Val Lys Ser Ser Lys Asp Phe
GCC ATG TGT TTT GGG AAG AAC TTC CCC AGG AAG AGC GAG GAG ATG CTC AAC CTC GTG AAG AGC AGC AAG GAC TTT

                                230                                   240                         250
Val Glu Asn Val Thr Ser Gly Asn Ala Val Asp Phe Phe Pro Val Leu Arg Tyr Leu Pro Asn Pro Ala Leu Lys
GTG GAG AAT GTC ACC TCA GGG AAT GCT GTG GAC TTC TTT CCG GTC CTG CGC TAC CTG CCC AAC CCA GCC CTC AAG

                                260                                   270
Arg Phe Lys Asn Phe Asn Asp Asn Phe Val Leu Ser Leu Gln Lys Thr Val Gln Glu His Tyr Gln Asp Phe Asn
AGG TTT AAG AAC TTC AAT GAT AAC TTT GTG CTG TCT CTG CAG AAA ACA GTC CAG GAA CAC TAT CAA GAC TTC AAC

                                280                                   290                         300
Lys Asn Ser Ile Gln Asp Ile Thr Gly Ala Leu Phe Lys His Ser Glu Asn Tyr Lys Asp Asn Gly Gly Leu Ile
AAG AAC AGT ATC CAG GAC ATC ACA GGC GCC CTG TTC AAG CAC AGT GAG AAC TAC AAA GAC AAC GGT GGT CTC ATC

                                310                                   320
Pro Gln Glu Lys Ile Val Asn Ile Val Asn Asp Ile Phe Gly Ala Gly Phe Glu Thr Val Thr Thr Ala Ile Phe
CCT CAG GAG AAG ATT GTC AAC ATT GTC AAT GAC ATC TTT GGA GCT GGA TTT GAA ACA GTC ACA ACA GCC ATC TTC

                                330                                   340                         350
Trp Ser Ile Leu Leu Leu Val Thr Glu Pro Lys Val Gln Arg Lys Ile His Glu Glu Leu Asp Thr Val Ile Gly
TGG AGC ATT TTG CTA CTT GTG ACA GAG CCC AAG GTG CAG AGG AAG ATT CAT GAG GAG CTG GAC ACG GTG ATT GGC

                                360                                   370
Arg Asp Arg Gln Pro Arg Leu Ser Asp Arg Pro Gln Leu Pro Tyr Leu Glu Ala Phe Ile Leu Glu Ile Tyr Arg
AGA GAT CGG CAG CCA CGG CTT TCT GAC AGA CCC CAG CTG CCA TAT CTG GAG GCC TTC ATC CTG GAG ATC TAC CGA

                                380                                   390                         400
Tyr Thr Ser Phe Val Pro Phe Thr Ile Pro His Ser Thr Thr Arg Asp Thr Ser Leu Asn Gly Phe His Ile Pro
TAC ACA TCC TTT GTC CCC TTC ACC ATC CCC CAC AGC ACA ACG AGG GAC ACC TCA CTG AAT GGC TTC CAC ATT CCC

                                410                                   420
Lys Glu Cys Cys Ile Phe Ile Asn Gln Trp Gln Val Asn His Asp Glu Lys Gln Trp Lys Asp Pro Phe Val Phe
AAG GAG TGC TGC ATC TTC ATA AAC CAG TGG CAG GTC AAC CAT GAT GAG AAG CAG TGG AAA GAC CCC TTT GTG TTC

                                430                                   440                         450
Arg Pro Glu Arg Phe Leu Thr Asn Asp Asn Thr Ala Ile Asp Lys Thr Leu Ser Glu Lys Val Met Leu Phe Gly
CGC CCA GAG CGG TTT CTT ACC AAT GAC AAC ACG GCC ATC GAC AAG ACC CTG AGT GAG AAG GTG ATG CTC TTC GGC

                                460                                   470
Leu Gly Lys Arg Arg Cys Ile Gly Glu Ile Pro Ala Lys Trp Glu Val Phe Leu Phe Leu Ala Ile Leu Leu His
TTG GGA AAG CGC CGG TGC ATT GCC GAG ATC CCG GCC AAG TGG GAA GTC TTC CTC TTC TTA GCC ATC CTC CTG CAT

                                480                                   490                         500
Gln Leu Glu Phe Thr Val Pro Pro Gly Val Lys Val Asp Leu Thr Pro Ser Tyr Gly Leu Thr Met Lys Pro Arg
CAG CTG GAG TTC ACT GTG CCA CCG GGC GTG AAG GTG GAC CTG ACA CCC AGC TAT GGG CTG ACC ATG AAG CCC AGA

                                510
Thr Cys Glu His Val Gln Ala Trp Pro Arg Phe Ser Lys
ACC TGT GAA CAC GTC CAG GCC TGG CCA CGC TTC TCC AAG TGA AGA TGG CCG AGA CAT CGG CCG CCA CCC TTG TTC

CTT TTC CTT TCT TTT TAA ATA ACA GCT TTT TCA AGA TAC AAT TCC TCC ACC ATT TAA TTC AGC TCC AAT CAA TTT

TCA ATA TTG TCT ACA CTG TTC CCT GCA AAC CCA TAC CCA TTA AGA TTT ATG ACT ATT CCT CCT ACC CTG TTT CGC

TTG CTG TGC CAC GTG CTA ATC TAG TTT TTG ACT CAA TAG ATT TGC CAA CTC TGG CTG - - -
```

FIG. 2. The coding nucleotides sequence of rat MC-inducible cytochrome P-450d cDNA and its corresponding amino acid sequence. The underlined amino acid sequence is the homologous region of various species of cytochrome P-450.

highly conserved throughout the various forms of P-450 sequences than HR1, we conclude that the cysteine in HR2 is most likely to be the fifth ligand to the heme of P-450 molecules. Haniu *et al.*, however, proposed that the cysteine residue in the HR1

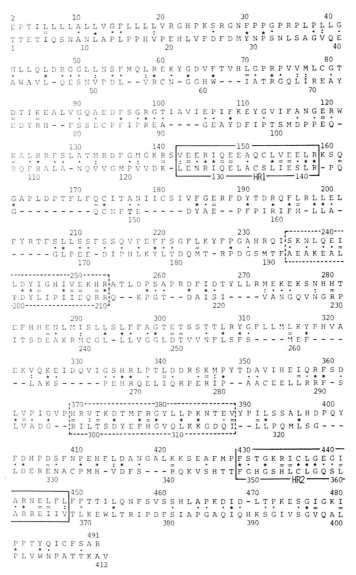

Fig. 3. Optimally matched alignment of P-450b and P-450cam sequences. The aligned amino acids are graded according to the value of the corresponding mutation data matrix element, mi,j (2) and indicated by the symbol between the single letter codes: $m \leq 0$ (blank); $m=1$ (.); $m=2$ (:); $m=3$ (=); $m \geq 4$ (*). Two highly homologous regions are enclosed in solid lines and labeled HR1 and HR2. Two other wealky homologous regions are shown in boxes with broken lines.

region of P-450cam functions as the fifth ligand to the heme on the basis of chemical modification with monoiodeacetamide. The cysteine residue in HR2 of P-450cam is the most reactive to the chemical of all eight cysteines in the P-450cam molecules. They claimed that this result lends supporting evidence against this cysteine being the 5th ligand to the heme and that the slowly reactive cysteine in HR1 is the most plausible ligand (15). These two alternatives should be decided experimentally.

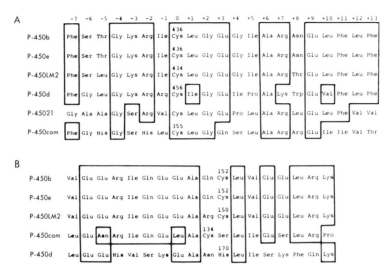

FIG. 4. Comparison of amino acid sequences of the homologous regions of various species of cytochrome P-450. We carried out a sequence comparison between five or six species of cytochrome P-450 as described previously (17). The amino acids contained in more than four species of cytochrome P-450 are enclosed by solid lines. A: HR2 region (see Fig. 3). B: HR1 (see Fig. 3).

When the two sequences of P-450b and -e are compared, fourteen amino acid replacements are found between them and occur in relatively limited portions of the molecules; these replacements are dispersed around the HR2 region. Because the catalytic activities of cytochrome P-450b and -e are clearly different from each other, at least some of these variable amino acids may take part in the interaction with substrates.

Genomic DNA Cloning and Its Structural Analysis

In order to quantitate the gene dosage of PB inducible cytochrome P-450 in rat haploid genome, Cot and Southern blot analyses were performed with the clone P-450h cDNA as a probe; these suggest the presence of approximately six genes or gene-like DNA sequences with homology to the cloned P-450 cDNA (22). In order to verify the multiplicity of PB-inducible cytochrome P-450 gene in the rat genome, we isolated genomic clones for the cytochrome by screening a rat gene library of Charon 4A with the cloned cDNA as a probe. After about 1×10^6 plaques were screened, nine recombinant phages which carried DNA sequences hybridizing with the cDNA were isolated and designated as pgP-450pb1 to 9. Since three of them (pgP-450pb2, 3 and 4) showed the same patterns of restriction cleavage and Southern blot analysis, we regarded these clones as identical. As shown in Fig. 5, pgP-450bp1 and 8 have an overlapping sequence with each other, and altogether they covered approximately 22 kb of the genomic DNA sequence. The other five genomic clones showed different restriction cleavage maps from one another, and from that of the one described above. Therefore, six independent genomic clones which showed sequence homology to the cloned P-450 cDNA were isolated, but this does not necessarily mean that all the isolated DNA sequences are

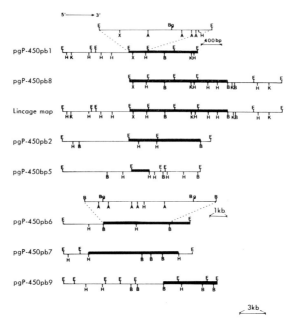

FIG. 5.   Restriction cleavage map of genomic clones. Bold lines show fragments hybridizable with P-450b cDNA. E, *Eco* RI; H, *Hind* III; B, *Bam* HI; K, *Kpn* 1; X, *Xba* I; A, *Ava* II; Bg, *Bgl* II.

true genes for PB-inducible P-450; some of them may be pseudogenes, as is often the case with other eukaryotic genes. Sequence analysis of these isolated DNAs is necessary to clarify these points.

One of the cloned genomic DNA, pgP-450pb6 was first chosen for sequence analysis because this clone contained a DNA insert that hybridized most strongly with the cDNA probe and was one of those most extended toward the 5′ direction of the gene. However, because this clone was found to lack the sequence of the 3′ end region of the cytochrome P-450 gene, we isolated another clone, pgP-450pb12, whose insert covers the missing sequence in pgP-450pb6 from the rat *Hae* III gene library (Fig. 6B).

We determined the nucleotide sequence of all exon and their flanking regions in the intron of a cytochrome P-450 gene as follows (23). Restriction fragments containing exon sequences were first identified by Southern blot analysis using the labeled cDNA as a probe and then appropriate restriction sites were chosen for end labeling by the method of Maxam and Gilbert. In most cases, restriction sites commonly found in both the cDNA and the genomic sequences were used. Finally, the exact coding nucleotide sequences in the exon and their flanking regions of the intervening sequences were determined in reference to the cDNA sequence and the consensus sequences of the exon-intron boundary (5). The general strategy for sequencing is depicted in Fig. 6C. 5′ end of the gene was determined to be an A, 30 bases upstream from the initiation codon by S1 nuclease protection mapping procedures. Twenty-seven bp further upstream from this A a possible modified TATA sequence, CATAAA, was found.

The poly(A) attachment site at the 3′end of the genomic sequence was assigned by comparison with the cDNA sequences which were determined from isolated cDNA

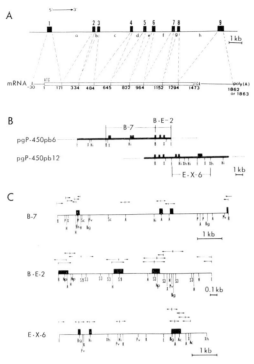

FIG. 6. Organization of rat PB-inducible cytochrome P-450 gene and strategy for its sequence analysis. A: the gene structure and its correspondence to the mRNA structure. Closed boxes indicate exon sequences numbered 1 to 9 and thin lines show intervening sequences (a–h). B: two genomic clones (pgP-450pb6 and -12) are arranged to show their overlapping DNA fragments. C: sequencing strategy of the cloned gene. Each arrow indicates the direction and length of the DNA fragment analyzed from appropriate restriction sites. E, *Eco* RI; X, *Xba* I; Hi, *Hin* dIII; B, *Bam* HI; P, *Pst* I; H, *Hin* fI; Bs, *Bst* NI; Sc, *Sac* I; Bg, *Bgl* II; Pv, *Pvu* II; A, *Ava* II; Hp, *Hpa* II; S9, *Sau* 96I; K, *Kpn* I; Xh, *Xho* I; Ac, *Acc* I.

clones, pcP-450pb1, -3, and -4. The entire 3′ trailer sequence of the messenger is encoded by exon 9, the last exon, together with the coding sequence for the COOH-terminal amino acids. Around 20 bp upstream from the poly(A) attachment site, no consensus poly(A) attachment signal AATAAA (24) is found, but a possible equivalent sequence, GGTAAA, is present 25 or 26 bp upstream from the poly(A) attachment site and this sequence is also found at the same position in the cDNA sequence, showing that this gene is actually transcribed into the mRNA.

The nucleotide sequences of all exons and their flanking regions in the introns thus determined are shown in Fig. 7, together with the two cDNA sequence for comparison.

On the whole the cytochrome P-450 gene is approximately 14 kb from the transcription-initiation site to the poly(A) attachment site and is separated into nine exons by eight intervening sequences. Except for the ninth (568 or 569 bp), all the exons are more or less similar in size, variyng from 150 bp for the third to 201 bp for the first; the sizes of the introns are much more variable, ranging from 0.3 to 3.2 kb. The boundary sequences of all eight introns agree with the consensus sequence for such

Y. FUJII-KURIYAMA ET AL.

TGAACATATGAAGTTGCATAACTGAGTGTAGGGGCAGATTCAGC<u>ATAAAA</u>GATCCTGCTGGAGAGCATGCACTGAAGTCTACCGTGGTTACACCAGGACC ATG GAG CCC AGT ATC

TTG CTC CTC CTT GCT CTC CTT GTG GGC TTC TTG TTA CTC TTA GTC AGG GGA CAC CCA AAG TCC CGT GGC AAC TTC CCA CCA GGA CCT CGT
--- ---
--- ---

CCC CTT CCC CTC TTG GGG AAC CTC CTG CAG TTG GAC AGA GGA GGC CTC CTC AAT TCC TTC ATG CAG GTGAGATATTCACAGGGCCTGGTGT-----
--- --- --- --- --- --- --- --- --- --- --- --- --G --- --- --- --- --- --- --- ---
--- --- --- --- --- --- --- --- --- --- --- --- --G --- --- --- --- --- --- --- ---

3.2 kb   -----CAGTCCTGTGCCTTTTAGTTTGCAG CTT CGC GAA AAA TAT GGA GAT GTG TTC ACA GTA CAC CTG GGA CCA AGG CCT GTG GTC A
                                       --- --A --- --- --- --- --- --- --- --- --- --- --- --- --- --- --- ---
                                       --- --A --- --- --- --- --- --- --- --- --- --- --- --- --- --- --- ---

TG CTA TGT GGG ACA GAC ACC ATA AAG GAG GCT CTG GTG GGC CAA GCT GAG GAT TTC TCT GGT CGG GGA ACA ATC GCT GTG ATT GAG CCA
-- ---
-- ---

ATC TTC AAG GAA TAT G GTAAGACTCTCAAAGGTTTGGGATG-----   0.3 kb   -----ATCCATGCTTCCCCTACTTTGTCAG GT GTG ATC TTT GCC AAT G
--- --- --- --- --- -   -- --- --- --- --- --- ---

GG GAA CGC TGG AAG GCC CTT CGG CGA TTC TCT CTG GCT ACC ATG AGA GAC TTT GGG ATG GGA AAG AGG AGT GTG GAA GAA CGG ATT CAG
-- ---
-- ---

GAG GAA GCC CAA TGT TTG GTG GAG GAA CTG CGG AAA TCC CAG G GTGAATCGGAAAGG-----   2.3 kb   -----CTCTTATCCTGCCTCCTCATCCTCC
--- --- --- --- --- --- --- --- --- --- --- --- --- --- -

AG GA GCC CCA CTG GAT CCC ACC TTC CTC TTC CAG TGC ATC ACA GCC AAC ATC ATC TGC TCC ATT GTG TTT GGA GAG CGC TTT GAC TAC A
-- ---

CA GAC CGC CAG TTC CTG CGC CTG TTG GAG CTG TTC TAC CGG ACC TTT TCC CTC CTA AGT TCA TTC TCC AGC CAG GTCCGTGGGTGGGAAGAGAA
-- ---

GAGTA-----   0.8 kb   -----TGAGGTGGTGGTTCTTGCCTTACAG GTG TTT GAG TTC TTC TCT GGG TTC CTG AAA TAC TTT CCT GGT GCC CAC AG
                                                            --- --- --- --- --- --- --- --- --- --- --- --- --- --- --- --

A CAA ATC TCC AAA AAC CTC CAG GAA ATC CTC GAT TAC ATT GGC CAT ATT GTG GAG AAG CAC AGG GCC ACC TTA GAC CCC AGC GCT CCA C
- --A --- --- ---
- --A --- --- ---

GA GAC TTC ATC GAC ACT TAC CTT CTG CGC ATG GAG AAG GTGAGTCCTGCATGGATGAGAGAGG-----   0.5 kb   -----CCATTCGCCCCCCAGGTGCAA
-- --- --- --- --- --- --- --- --- --- --- --- ---

CCAG GAG AAG TCG AAC CAC CAC ACA GAG TTC CAT CAT GAG AAC CTC ATG ATC TCC CTG CTC TCT CTC TTC TTT GCT GGC ACT GAG ACC GG
--- --A-
--- --A-

C AGC ACC ACA CTC CGC TAT GGT TTC CTG CTC ATG CTC AAG TAC CCC CAT GTC ACA G GTATATCATGGGGGGTACCGTTGG-----   1.6 kb   --
- --- --- --- --- --- --- --- --- --- --- --- --G --- --- --- --- --- --- G-- -

---CCCTTTCTCGCAG TG AAA GTC CAA AAG GAG ATT GAT CAG GTG ATT GGC TCT CAC AGG CCA TCA TCC CTT GAT GAT CGT ACC AAA ATG CCA
                A-- --- --- --- --- --- --- --- --- --- --- --C --- --A --- C-- -T- --- A-- --- --- --C --C -GT --- ---

TAC ACT GAT GCA GTC ATC CAC GAG ATT CAG AGG TTT GCA GAT CTT GCC CCA ATT GGT TTA CCA CAC AGA GTC ACC AAA GAC ACC ATG TTC
--- --- --- --- --- --T --- --- --- --- --- --- --- --- --- --- --- --- --- T-- --- --- -T- --T --- --A G-- --- --- ---

CGA GGG TAC CTG CTC CCC AAG GTGAGGCCAACCCGTGAATTCCGCGA-----   0.3 kb   -----AACATCTTATCTATAACTCTCCCAG AAC ACT GAG GTG T
--- --- --- --- --T --- ---   --- --- --A --- -

AT CCC ATC CTG AGT TCA GCT CTC CAT GAC CCA CAG TAC TTT GAC CAT CCA GAC ACC TTC AAT CCT GAG CAC TTC CTG GAT GCC GAT GGG
-C --- --- --- --- --- --- --- --- --- --- --C --- --- G-- --- --- --- --- --- --A --- --- --- --- --- A-- ---

ACA CTG AAA AAG AGT GAA GCT TTT ATG CCC TTC TCC ACA G GTGAGGCAGAATTGTGATTCCTTT-----   3.2 kb   -----AGCATGTCACTCTCTTGGT
G-- --- --- --- --- --- --C --- --- --- --- -

CAG GA AAG CGC ATT TGT CTT GGC GAA GGC ATT GCC CGA AAT GAA TTG TTC CTC TTC TTC ACC ACC ATC CTC CAG AAC TTC TCT GTG TCA
-- ---

AGC CAT TTG GCT CCC AAG GAC ATT GAC CTC ACG CCC AAG GAG AGT GGC ATT GGA AAA ATA CCT CCA ACG TAC CAG ATC TGC TTC TCA GCT
--- ---

CGG TGA TCCGGCTGAGGCAGCCATGTGCCCCAGTTCTGTTGGGAATGGCCTCATGTTTCTGCCTCTGGGGGACCTGCTGAAAACCAGGCTCCAAGGCCACTGCTCCACATCTTCCTA
--- --- -----------------G---

TTGCAGTTCTCCAAAGTCCCAAGGCTTTTCTTATTCCTGTGAATGGCACTGAAGAAGTCAATCGGCTGTCTTATTTTGACATGTGACAGAGATTTCATGAGTCCACATCTCATGCTGA

GTTACTTCCCTCTTCCTCCTAACAGCCCATGTCCCCAGTTATCAGCCCTCCATGGTCTGTGATCTGTGCTAATGGACTCTGTATATGGTCTCAGTGCTCTATGTCTACAGAGACTTACATAGT

ATGTATGGTTCAGGTAAACAGAATCACAGAGTGTGTGA GCTTCGGTGTCTGTGCCTTTACTTCACATAATATTATTCTAGGTTCCTGTGTTGTTCTACAGGCCACAGTCACACACATTCAT

FIG. 7. Nucleotide sequence of PB-inducible cytochrome P-450 gene and comparison with the cDNA sequences. Nucleotide sequences corresponding to all nine exons and their franking regions in the intervening sequences were determined as described in Fig. 6 and are shown on the upper line. The 5′ end of the gene was assigned by S1 mapping procedure and the poly(A) attachment site was determined by comparison with the cDNA sequence; these are indicated by arrows. The cDNA sequences determined from pcP-450pb2 (P-450e cDNA) and from pcP-450pb1, -3, and -4 (P-450b cDNA) are shown in the middle and lower lines, respectively. Dashes show absence of nucleotide substitution from the upper genomic sequence.

regions (5). Each intron begins with G-T-C at the 5′ terminus and ends with A-G at the 3′ terminus.

As compared in detail with the cDNA sequences, the genomic sequence determined here is consistent with that of pcP-450pb2, except for the neutral base substitutions at the third positions of codons 49, 59, and 258. A recent report from Yuan *et al.* who analyzed about 75% of the amino acid sequences of their two purified cytochrome P-450s, shows that the sequence of pcP-450pb1 and -4 is for cytochrome P-450b, a major form of PB-inducible cytochrome P-450, and that of pcP-450pb2 is for cytochrome P-450e, a minor form of a PB-inducible one (26). Therefore, we assume that the genomic sequence determined here is for the cytochrome P-450e gene, when allelic polymorphism and possible sequencing errors are taken into consideration. On the other hand, a considerable number of base substitutions are observed between the sequences of this gene and pcP-450pb1 and -4 (cytochrome P-450b cDNA). Forty base substitutions were found in the sequence of approximately 1,900 bases examined and 15 of them result in 14 amino acid replacements. It should be noted that these substitutions occur in relatively limited regions of the sequences. Most of them are found in exons 6, 7, 8, and 9 but most frequently in exon 7. We recently completed the nucleotide sequence of the cytochrome P-450b gene; its general structure is very similar to that of the cytochrome P-450e gene in numbers of exons and introns and their relative locations except that the first intron (12 kb) of cytochrome P-450b gene is much longer than that (3.6 kb) of cytochrome P-450e gene. The P-450b gene, therefore, is much longer (approximately 23 kb) than the P-450e gene (Suwa *et al.* unpublished observation). Cytochrome P-450b is a more abundant species than P-450e in the livers of PB-treated rats. A detailed comparison of the structures of these two cytochrome P-450 genes will provide a clue to the DNA element(s) governing quantitative regulation of the cytochrome in drug-treated animals.

In contrast to the genes of PB-inducible cytochrome P-450, there appears to be a limited number of genes for MC-inducible P-450 in rat haploid genome. In Southern blot analysis using cloned P-450d cDNA as a probe, each of *Eco* RI, *Bam* HI, and *Hin* dIII digestion of rat DNA gave only two hybridization bands, suggesting the presence of at least two genes for MC-inducible P-450. We have isolated two independent genomic clones of MC-inducible P-450 from a rat gene library using cloned P-450d cDNA as a probe, and a partial sequence analysis of these cloned genes revealed that one is for cytochrome P-450d and the other for cytochrome P-450c (Sogawa *et al.*, unpublished observations). The two forms of cytochrome P-450 were purified from livers of MC-treated rats and analyzed in an N-terminal sequence of about 20 amino acids (4). Sequence analysis of these genomic clones is now underway and will provide generous information on the regulatory DNA sequence in the promoter region and molecular evolution of the genes.

REFERENCES

1. Adesnik, M., Bar Nun, S., Mashio, F., Zunich, M., Lipman, A., and Bard, E. Mechanism of induction of cytochrome P-450. *J. Biol. Chem.*, **256**, 10340–10345 (1981).
2. Barker, W. C. and Dayhoff, M. O. *In* "Atlas of Protein Sequence and Structure," ed.

M. O. Dayhoff, Vol. 5, pp. 101–110 (1972). National Biomedical Research Foundation, Silver Spring.

3. Botelho, L. H., Ryan, D. E., and Levin, W. Amino acid composition and partial amino acid sequences of these highly purified forms of liver microsomal cytochrome P-450 from rats treated with polychlorinated biphenyls, phenobarbital, or 3-methylcholanthrene. *J. Biol. Chem.*, **254**, 5635–5640 (1979).

4. Botelho, L. H., Ryan, D. E., Yuan, P.-M., Kutny, R., Shively, J. E., and Levin, W. Amino-terminal and carboxy-terminal sequence of hepatic microsomal cytochrome P-450d, a unique hemoprotein from rats treated with isosafrole. *Biochemistry*, **21**, 1152–1155 (1982).

5. Breathnach, R. and Chambon, P. Organization and expression of eukaryotic split genes coding for proteins. *Annu. Rev. Biochem.*, **50**, 349–383 (1981).

6. Colbert, R. A., Bresnick, E., Levin, W., Ryan, D. E., and Thomas, P. E. Synthesis of liver cytochrome P-450b in a cell-free protein synthesizing system. *Biochem. Biophys. Res. Commun.*, **91**, 886–891 (1979).

7. Dubois, R. N. and Waterman, M. R. Effect of phenobarbital administration to rats on the level of the *in vitro* synthesis of cytochrome P-450 directed by total rat liver RNA. *Biochem. Biophys. Res. Commun.*, **90**, 150–157 (1979).

8. Dus, K., Litchfield, W. J., Minguel, A. G., Hoeven, T. A., Haugen, D. A., Dean, W. L., and Coon, M. J. Structural resemblance of cytochrome P-450 isolated from *Pseudomonas putida* and from rabbit liver microsomes. *Biochem. Biophys. Res. Commun.*, **60**, 15–21 (1974).

9. Fujii-Kuriyama, Y., Taniguchi, T., Mizukami, Y., Sakai, M., Tashiro, Y., and Muramatsu, M. Construction and identification of a hybrid plasmid containing DNA sequence complementary to phenobarbital-inducible cytochrome P-450 messenger RNA from rat liver. *J. Biochem.*, **89**, 1869–1879 (1981).

10. Fujii-Kuriyama, Y., Mizukami, Y., Kawajiri, K., Sogawa, K., and Muramatsu, M. Primary structure of a cytochrome P-450: coding nucleotide sequence of phenobarbital-inducible cytochrome P-450 cDNA from rat liver. *Proc. Natl. Acad. Sci. U. S.*, **79**, 2793–2797 (1982).

11. Gotoh, O., Tagashira, Y., Iizuka, T., and Fujii-Kuriyama, Y. Structural characteristics of cytochrome P-450. Possible location of the heme-binding cytochrome in determined amino acid sequences. *J. Biochem.*, **93**, 807–817 (1983).

12. Guengerich, F. P. Isolation and purification of cytochrome P-450, and the existence of multiple forms. *Pharmacol. Ther.*, **6**, 99–121 (1979).

13. Gunsalus, I. C. and Sligar, S. G. Oxygen reduction by the P-450 monooxygenase systems. *Adv. Enzymol.*, **47**, 1–44 (1978).

14. Haniu, M., Armes, L. G., Yasunobu, K. T., Shastry, B. A., and Gunsalus, I. C. Amino acid sequence of *Pseudomonas putida* cytochrome P-450. II. Cyanogen bromide peptides, acid cleavage peptide, and the complete sequence. *J. Biol. Chem.*, **257**, 12664–12671 (1982).

15. Haniu, M., Shively, J. E., and Hall, P. F. Structural studies on the steroid-hydroxylase cytochrome P-450 from porcine adrenal gland. *Fed. Proc.*, **42**, 1774 (1983).

16. Haniu, M., Yasunobu, K. T., and Gunsalus, I. C. Heme binding and substrate-protected cysteine residues in P-450 cam. *Biochem. Biophys. Res. Commun.*, **116**, 30–38 (1983).

17. Kawajiri, K., Gotoh, O., Sogawa, K., Tagashira, Y., Muramatsu, M., and Fujii-Kuriyama, Y. Coding nucleotide sequence of 3-methylcholanthrene-inducible cytochrome P-450d cDNA from rat liver. *Proc. Natl. Acad. Sci. U. S.*, **81**, 1649–1653 (1984).

18. Kamataki, T., Maeda, K., Yamazoe, Y., Matsuda, N., Ishii, K., and Kato, R. A high-spin form of cytochrome P-450, highly purified from polychlorinated biphenyl-treated

rats. Catalytic characterization and immunochemical quantitation in liver microsomes. *Mol. Pharmacol.*, **24**, 146–155 (1983).

19. Kawajiri, K., Sogawa, K., Gotoh, O., Tagashira, Y., Muramatsu, M., and Fujii-Kuriyama, Y. Molecular cloning of a complementary DNA to 3-methylcholanthrene-inducible cytochrome P-450 mRNA from rat liver. *J. Biochem.*, **94**, 1465–1473 (1983).

20. Kawajiri, K., Yonekawa, H., Harada, N., Noshiro, M., Omura, T., and Tagashira, Y. Immunochemical study on the role of different types of microsomal cytochrome P-450 in mutagenesis by chemical carcinogens. *Cancer Res.*, **40**, 1652–1657 (1980).

21. Lu, A.Y.H. and West, S. B. Multiplicity of mammalian microsomal cytochromes P-450. *Pharmacol. Rev.*, **31**, 227–295 (1980).

22. Mizukami, Y., Fujii-Kuriyama, Y., and Muramatsu, M. Multiplicity of deoxyribonucleic acid sequences with homology to a closed complementary deoxyribonucleic acid coding for rat phenobarbital-inducible cytochrome P-450. *Biochemistry*, **22**, 1223–1229 (1983).

23. Mizukami, Y., Sogawa, K., Suwa, Y., Muramatsu, M., and Fujii-Kuriyama, Y. Gene structure of a phenobarbital-inducible cytochrome P-450 in rat liver. *Proc. Natl. Acad. Sci. U. S.*, **80**, 3958–3962 (1983).

24. Proudfoot, N. J. and Brownlee, G. G. 3′Non-coding region sequences in eukaryotic messenger RNA. *Nature*, **263**, 211–214 (1976).

25. Sato, R. and Omura, T. eds. "Cytochrome P-450" (1978). Kodansha, Tokyo/Academic Press, New York.

26. Yuan, P.M., Ryan, D. E., Levin, W., and Shively, J. E. Identification and localization of amino acid substitutions between two phenobarbital-inducible rat hepatic microsomal cytochrome P-450 by microsequence analysis. *Proc. Natl. Acad. Sci. U. S.*, **80**, 1169–1173 (1983).

AUTHOR INDEX

SUBJECT INDEX